Cooking
Healthy with a
Pressure
Cooker

Also by JoAnna M. Lund

Cooking Healthy with a Pressure Cooker

A HEALTHY EXCHANGES® COOKBOOK

JoAnna M. Lund

with
Barbara Alpert

A Perigee Book

A PERIGEE BOOK
Published by the Penguin Group
Penguin Group (USA) Inc.
375 Hudson Street, New York, New York 10014, USA
Penguin Group (Canada), 90 Eglinton Avenue East, Suite 700, Toronto, Ontario M4P 2Y3, Canada
(a division of Pearson Penguin Canada Inc.)
Penguin Books Ltd., 80 Strand, London WC2R 0RL, England
Penguin Group Ireland, 25 St. Stephen's Green, Dublin 2, Ireland (a division of Penguin Books Ltd.)
Penguin Group (Australia), 250 Camberwell Road, Camberwell, Victoria 3124, Australia
(a division of Pearson Australia Group Pty. Ltd.)
Penguin Books India Pvt. Ltd., 11 Community Centre, Panchsheel Park, New Delhi—110 017, India
Penguin Group (NZ), 67 Apollo Drive, Rosedale, North Shore 0632, New Zealand
(a division of Pearson New Zealand Ltd.)
Penguin Books (South Africa) (Pty.) Ltd., 24 Sturdee Avenue, Rosebank, Johannesburg 2196,
South Africa

Penguin Books Ltd., Registered Offices: 80 Strand, London WC2R 0RL, England

While the author has made every effort to provide accurate telephone numbers and Internet addresses at
the time of publication, neither the publisher nor the author assumes any responsibility for errors, or for
changes that occur after publication. Further, the publisher does not have any control over and does not
assume any responsibility for author or third-party websites or their content.

For more information about Healthy Exchanges products, contact:
Healthy Exchanges, Inc.
P.O. Box 80
DeWitt, IA 52742-0080
(563) 659-8234
www.HealthyExchanges.com

First edition: December 2007

Library of Congress Cataloging-in-Publication Data

Lund, JoAnna M.
    Cooking healthy with a pressure cooker : a Healthy Exchanges cookbook / JoAnna M. Lund with
Barbara Alpert.
        p.   cm.
    Includes index.
    ISBN 978-0-399-53375-4
    1. Pressure cookery. 2. Reducing diets—Recipes. 3. Diabetes—Diet therapy—Recipes. I. Alpert,
Barbara.   II. Title.

TX840.P7L86 2007
641.5'87—dc22

2007013115

PRINTED IN THE UNITED STATES OF AMERICA

10   9   8   7   6   5   4   3   2   1

PUBLISHER'S NOTE: The recipes contained in this book are to be followed exactly as written. The
publisher is not responsible for your specific health or allergy needs that may require medical supervi-
sion. The publisher is not responsible for any adverse reactions to the recipes contained in this book.

Most Perigee Books are available at special quantity discounts for bulk purchases for sales promotions,
premiums, fund-raising, or educational use. Special books, or book excerpts, can also be created to fit
specific needs. For details, write: Special Markets, Penguin Group (USA) Inc., 375 Hudson Street, New
York, New York 10014.

Dedication

This book is dedicated in loving memory, as all of my books are, to my parents, Jerome and Agnes McAndrews. My mother had the inspiring ability to feed our family well by taking often very basic ingredients and transforming them into delicious meals that satisfied the soul as well as the tummy. She used her infinite knowledge of the foods available to her, along with the few appliances she had (including her pressure cooker), to create dishes that she was proud to serve to anyone sharing our table. And I know my father admired the practicality of that old pressure cooker as well as her creativity in using it.

I hope you enjoy using your much-improved pressure cooker to prepare the recipes in this book. I give much of the credit for their creation to my parents, from whom I inherited both my mother's artistic talents and my father's practical traits.

My mother always found a few minutes in a very busy day to write her beautiful poems. This is one I have always liked and hope you will, too.

The Clock of Life

Life
  is like one fleeting hour—
  here for sixty precious minutes.
Each second fills the heart
  with sunshine, joy and even bitter pain
  which we all cherish unto the end.
When the clock strikes,
  the hour at last has come and with strained ears
  we listen for the last stroke.
So like our lives,
  then all is silent—
  and only the Master can determine the time.

—Agnes Carrington McAndrews

Acknowledgments

While the pressure cooker certainly cuts down on cooking time, getting these recipes right took plenty of help from a lot of people. For helping "relieve the pressure," so to speak, I want to thank:

Shirley Morrow, Rita Ahlers, Phyllis Bickford, Cheryl Hageman, Gina Griep, and Jean Martens—my employees. They all did what they do best—and together we got it done. Whether it was typing recipes or stirring up some new dishes, cleaning the kitchen or handling the busy phones, they helped me do what I do best, and I thank them all!

Cliff Lund—my husband. Cliff is a great believer in not letting the pressure get to you, and he kept me going when I wasn't sure I'd find the energy to do it all. Even when he was on the road truckin', he called me several times every day to check in and make sure I was hanging in there. And he was always ready to taste another dish—no matter how many he had tried that day!

Barbara Alpert—my writing partner. She knows what pressure feels like—she's a teacher in addition to working with me on my books. She helps take the pressure off me by making suggestions that always make my books better!

Coleen O'Shea—my literary agent. No one is as cool under pressure as she is, which makes her a terrific partner in all my publishing activities. She listens to my ideas and helps me find a way to make them happen, even the ones that take extra effort!

John Duff—my publisher and editor. He doesn't pressure anyone to do something, just has a wonderful way of asking for this or that—and no one ever wants to say no to him!

God—my Creator and Savior. With His help and guidance, I handled the pressure of juggling work and family, taking care of my health, and finding time to do what I love, like working in my gardens. With His love, I was able to find the strength to finish this book.

Contents

Handling the Pressures of a Busy Life

C an you think of anyone who doesn't have loads of responsibilities, lots to do, and rarely enough time to do it all without feeling overwhelmed? I can't. The weight of all those responsibilities,
the feeling that your juggling act is about to come tumbling down
on your head, often goes hand in hand with excess weight and
other health concerns. So finding a way to handle the pressure better is a good idea—and it might just be the key to helping you live
a longer, better, and healthier life.

Take a moment and grab a calculator if you have one. Figure
out how many meals you prepare each day, then multiply that by
seven for the total in a week. Multiply that number by fifty weeks
a year (I'm hoping you get two weeks' vacation where you don't
have to do all the cooking!). Now take that number and multiply
it by the number of years you've been making meals for your
family.

Shocking, isn't it? No wonder you feel exhausted much of the
time. And wait, I didn't even have you add up the additional hours
of food shopping and preparation, not to mention the time you
spend on other housekeeping duties!

That's why I'm such a great believer in whatever makes meal
preparation faster, easier, and healthier. For me, that means choosing smart kitchen appliances and using healthy convenience foods
in my recipes. Anyone who does all that cooking needs *help*—and

I'm happy to report that, with this cookbook, the help you need is here.

But wait a minute. Your kitchen counters are already crowded with microwaves, food processors, electric double-sided grills, and more. Do you really *need* a pressure cooker?

That's up to you, of course. The fact that you're holding this cookbook tells me that you've already got one (as a wedding or shower gift, perhaps) or that you're planning to purchase one any day now. But maybe you're wondering if you'll use it. Does it deserve the space it's going to take up in your kitchen?

I think it does. But I didn't always think so.

Way Back When

When I was growing up back in the early 1950s, my mother used her pressure cooker a lot. We grew loads of fruits and vegetables in our garden, and she used it primarily for canning summer's bounty, so we could enjoy those veggies and fruits all year long. We didn't own a freezer and our refrigerator was relatively small, so Mom needed to find a way to store food for later use. Her pressure cooker was the answer! She also used it to turn inexpensive and tough meats into delicious and satisfying meals.

But one summer day, when I was about eight years old, I learned that this handy appliance wasn't always reliable. That night, the pressure cooker splashed Mom's supper onto the ceiling!

My younger sister and I had been playing in our clubhouse (actually a primitive tree house in a huge maple tree). It was a perfect late July day, about five in the afternoon. Mom was in the kitchen getting supper ready for our father, who would soon be returning from the Farmall factory (where he worked on the assembly line putting metal wheels on International Harvester tractors). Suddenly we heard a strange noise from inside the house and climbed down to see what it was.

My sister and I ran into the kitchen and saw that our mother was crying. She not only had a big mess to clean up, but she also didn't have much on hand to prepare another meal. I think we had to eat cheese sandwiches that night, and from that day on, I had a less idealistic opinion of this kitchen helper. While pressure cookers were a godsend for canning and preparing inexpensive meats, they also had a nasty reputation for exploding!

Now, flash forward to the early 1970s, when I was a young farm wife with three kids under the age of six. Those were not good times for farmers, so like many other farm wives, I got a job in town. I had to leave the house by 7 A.M. to get the kids to their babysitter. Then I'd drive forty-five miles to get to the bank where I worked, put in eight hours running a bookkeeping and proof machine, drive back to the babysitter to pick up the kids, and finally get home around 6 P.M. I had hungry kids and a husband who had worked out in the fields all day, so I had to get supper on the table fast! The pressure cooker I had received as a wedding gift became my best friend.

Even if I'd forgotten to take something out of the freezer that morning, I could have tasty soups and stews on the table in less than thirty minutes. Okay, my pressure cooker still exploded occasionally. (Just ask my daughter, Becky, and son James! I know they remember playing on the screened porch late one Saturday afternoon while I was canning applesauce in the kitchen. When that pressure cooker exploded, and the applesauce and glass jars flew all over the room, their eyes got as big as saucers. They loved my canned applesauce, and they were more upset that they wouldn't be having it anytime soon than they were about the mess. I, on the other hand, was upset that all my hard work had ended up on the ceiling, the floor, and the stove!)

Making the Case for These "Newfangled" Pressure Cookers

But oh, how times have changed. We're well into the twenty-first century, and the pressure cookers of today are as safe to use as a saucepan!

I can proudly say I have two new pressure cookers that I dearly love. I've even seen some electric pressure cookers that I'd love to try, but I just haven't been able to convince Cliff that I need another one! As much as he enjoys the foods I prepare in them, he keeps saying, "Where are you going to store it?"

That said, his eyes light up every time he sees a pressure cooker on my stove because he *knows* he's going to get something really good for supper!

So, if you don't already own an up-to-date pressure cooker, I highly recommend putting one on your birthday or holiday gift list. Maybe getting yet another kitchen appliance feels like a luxury, but bringing home something that helps you serve and eat healthier meals isn't an "extra"—it really can be a necessity!

Here's another reason that pressure cookers may be even more popular today than they were in the late '40s and early '50s. It brings together the strengths of two of our favorite appliances: It combines the speed of the microwave with the all-day comforting tastes produced by a slow cooker! So it allows the busy home cook to spend *minutes* in food preparation but produces a meal that tastes as if it took *hours*. Because foods cook faster at higher temperatures—using pressure to increase the temperature without burning the food—you can have a beef stew ready in twenty minutes or less, compared to hours of cooking on the stovetop or baking in the oven.

I can promise you that if you are just finding out about this great kitchen tool, you are going to be in for a world of good eating. You may be a bit afraid the first time you use it—but once you give it a try and get nothing but compliments from the lucky diners, you'll be sold on the pressure cooker every bit as much as I am!

Remember, the pressure cookers of today are not the same as the ones our mothers had in the 1950s and '60s. The modern versions have safety features built into them so that the chance of supper landing on the kitchen ceiling is almost nonexistent. The pressure cookers of today have had the fear factors removed; current models offer everything from easy locking lids to "blowout gaskets," which allow steam to release if the pressure gets too high, making those terrifying kitchen explosions a thing of the past. They are also much quieter than they used to be—so now, the only sound you'll hear is a gentle hissing as the pressure cooker cooks supper.

Turn on your favorite home-shopping channel, and you'll see that they're featuring pressure cookers as a kitchen "best bet" for the twenty-first century. In fact, the Cook's Essentials line at QVC includes both a manual and an electric version, and both turn up often in the station's cooking shows.

One woman recently told me she owns three pressure cookers, and added that she uses one of them at least two or three times a week. It is her favorite kitchen appliance. She's not alone. When I Googled "pressure cooker" on the Internet, I found more than 500,000 sites devoted to this astonishing appliance. Many of the sites shared a variety of recipes for the pressure cooker, but I didn't spot any specifically for people with diabetes, those with heart and cholesterol concerns, or those following a nationally known weight-loss program. So I decided to fill that need with this new cookbook, brimming with recipes that focus on ease of preparation, taste appeal, and common health concerns.

Feeling the Pressure, Letting It Go

Now, as long as we're talking about pressure, I wanted to share with you some thoughts I've had recently about how feeling the pressure in our everyday lives can be detrimental, and why I feel it's important to do something about that.

Think for a moment about how it feels to be under pressure—because of work, family problems, money worries, or health concerns. Your blood pressure increases, your heart has to work harder, your breathing is more labored, your concentration is poor, and your overall ability to live your life well is in real jeopardy.

If you spend too much time under that kind of tension, you may experience more physical symptoms, from aches and pains to panic attacks. It's a case of your emotions putting your health at greater risk. So, what can you do about it?

Change your focus.

Instead of focusing on the pressure wearing you down, choose to focus on something that makes you feel good. For me, the best pressure release I know is working in my gardens. There's so much to do, I can't think about anything else but what needs weeding, what needs picking, where I should place the flowers I've just picked, and what I might cook with the beautiful bounty from my tomato patch or fruit trees!

Even if I'm having a difficult week, digging in the dirt seems to push away all my worries and make me feel like a kid again. It's been my pressure release all my life, and I know it's sustained me during difficult times. Even when I didn't feel strong enough to wield a garden tool, I could sit on one of my benches and meditate on the glorious profusion of plants and trees that are a celebration of life in every leaf and bloom!

Help someone who may be under more pressure than you are.

Why would I suggest you find someone who needs help when you are already swamped by your own life? I've discovered that even the busiest people can make time for what makes them feel good. Can you do something, even something small, to take the pressure off someone else? My friend Barbara keeps an eye (and an ear) out for parents on the bus or subway whose babies or toddlers are being fussy. "I try to distract and entertain the kids for a few minutes, giving the parents a little break," she told me. She's taught more than a few little ones to stick out their tongues and wiggle their feet! She enjoys doing it, and everyone in the subway car appreciates the fact that the child is no longer wailing.

By looking for opportunities to alleviate the stress and tension someone else is struggling with, you set aside some of your own— at least for a while. It's a healthy choice to ease the pressure for another person . . . which has the surprising power to lessen your own.

Consider that maybe what you experience as pressure is actually a push to do better, be more, go further than you thought you could.

Learning something new is hard. Going outside your comfort zone is uncomfortable. Risking change can be unnerving. But it's also the only way to grow as a human being. Whether you decide to study a language or try wood carving, take salsa lessons or go back to school in your golden years, or just take on something new at the office, you may feel the pressure weighing on you, and think it would be easier to say no, to skip it, to stay home, to sit it out. But that kind of pressure stimulates the brain; provides excitement after a long stretch of same-old, same-old; and possibly points you down a path that will transform your life in a wonderful way.

If you've always dreamed of starting a business but everyone says it will be too hard, you could listen to the naysayers—or you could take a giant risk and test yourself. Change isn't easy, but it's how we as a species have evolved into the incredibly complex beings we are today. Let's keep pushing the limits of what we can do; I believe we'll discover that "pressure" is the route we must take to fulfill our most remarkable dreams!

Jo Anna

Please note:

In many of my cookbooks, I've included my Healthy Exchanges eating plan, which explains how to use my version of the "exchange" system for planning what to eat and how much to eat for optimum health and weight loss (or maintenance). Because this is a "special interest" cookbook, I've chosen to focus just on the recipes in this volume. If this is your first Healthy Exchanges cookbook, please check one of my other books for an explanation of the exchange system and an abundance of healthy cooking tips! Good choices include *The Open Road Cookbook* or *Cooking Healthy with Splenda*.

My Best Pressure Cooker Tips for Success

(I shared a version of these in my earlier book *JoAnna's Kitchen Miracles*.)

1. Whether you've just purchased a new pressure cooker or are now pulling your old one out of the back closet to use, I want you to read and practice three things from the instruction booklet before you start cooking anything in that pot!

   • Carefully read how to lock the lid correctly for cooking—and then do it.

   • Read how to know when your pressure cooker has reached the various pressure settings. Some have three (5 pounds—10 pounds—15 pounds) and others have only one. I suggest you fill it halfway with water. Watch and write down how long it takes to get to the various settings. I know you think you'll remember, but trust me, solid written notes are much more accurate than fading memories!

   • Read how to reduce the pressure on your cooker and how to unlock the lid. The water in that pot will work just fine for this practice session, also.

2. No matter what size pressure cooker you have, they tend to work best when they are at least halfway but no more than two-thirds filled. If this is more than you'll be able to use for one meal, the foods prepared in a pressure cooker almost always freeze beautifully. Cook once and eat twice—or more!

3. Because almost no steam escapes while cooking, you'll find that pressure cooker recipes require much less liquid than they would if cooked in a conventional saucepan. These recipes have already taken that into consideration. After you've prepared mine for a while, if you're ready to try to adapt your own recipes, look for similar recipes in this book and see how much liquid I used.

4. *Cooking time starts when the pressure is reached.* You start counting the time for cooking when the pressure called for in the recipe is reached, not from when you first put the cooker on the stove. I set my kitchen timer and find it works great. Even when I'm busy doing something else, that *ding* from the timer reminds me to get back to my pressure cooker.

5. When storing your pressure cooker, put the lid on upside down or lean it against the side of the pan. Here's why: If you lock the lid in place, the aroma from your last dish may still be wafting out of the pan when you take the lid off because there's no way for it to escape into the air!

6. Be careful when cooking foamy foods in your pressure cooker, as they could block the steaming vent. Applesauce, cranberries, rhubarb, oatmeal, rice, split peas, and pearl barley are the main culprits.

7. Along those lines, always make sure the vent pipe is clear before closing the lid. You can easily check this by holding the lid up to the light and looking through the vent. If it is blocked, you can clean it with a wooden toothpick. Why must it be clear? If the vent pipe is clogged, pressure may build up to unsafe levels.

8. *Never, never, never* open the pressure cooker when it is still under pressure! Always check the indicator or gently push the pressure regulator and listen for that hissing steam noise. If you can hear it, *don't* open the lid. If you can't hear the hiss, it's safe to take the lid off.

9. Once a year, check the rubber gasket to see if it has become hard or, the other extreme, soft and sticky. If either happens, it's time to replace it. The sealing gasket usually does not become soft unless it comes in constant contact with fat or oil. So, if you're using only my recipes, you shouldn't have to worry about this at all!

10. Be extra careful never to hit or bump the rim of the pressure cooker with a spoon or other cooking utensil because you could cause a small dent, which might prevent the pressure cooker from pressuring properly. (Even though I know this well, I have to remind myself not to do it!) When using a pressure cooker, keep the kids and spouse out of the kitchen if possible so you don't become distracted and accidentally "bruise" your pot. (Another good reason for keeping the kitchen off-limits during cooking is that you need to be able to hear the timer go off when it's time to remove the pressure cooker from the burner.)

Please note: We used an Innova brand 8-quart pressure cooker to test the recipes in this book.

A Peek Into My Healthy Exchanges Pantry

I do almost all of my shopping at a supermarket in my small town of DeWitt, Iowa. If I can't find an ingredient there, I don't use it in my recipes. I want you to be able to make any and all of these dishes without struggling to locate a particular ingredient. That's what it means to cook *The Healthy Exchanges Way*.

That said, I have tested brands from many different manufacturers, looking for the healthiest, tastiest, and easiest, to get items that deliver the most flavor for the least amount of fat, sugar, or calories. I update this list for every cookbook and for my newsletter readers every year in the March issue. If you find others you like as well *or better*, please use them. This is only a guide to make shopping and cooking easier for you.

Here are my preferred ingredients and brands, as of this time:

Egg substitute—*Egg Beaters*
Fat-free plain yogurt—*Dannon*
Nonfat dry milk powder—*Carnation*
Evaporated fat-free milk—*Carnation*
Fat-free milk
Fat-free cottage cheese
Fat-free cream cheese—*Philadelphia*
Fat-free half & half—*Land O Lakes*
Fat-free mayonnaise—*Kraft*

Fat-free dressings—*Kraft*

No-fat sour cream—*Land O Lakes*

"Diet" margarine—*I Can't Believe It's Not Butter! Light*

Cooking sprays

Olive oil– and butter-flavored—*Pam*

Butter-flavored, for spritzing *after* cooking—*I Can't Believe It's Not Butter!*

Cooking oil—*Puritan Canola Oil*

Reduced-calorie whipped topping—*Cool Whip Lite* or *Free*

White sugar substitute—*Splenda*

Baking mix—*Bisquick Heart Smart*

Quick oats—*Quaker*

Graham cracker crumbs—*Nabisco Honey Maid*

Sugar-free pancake syrup—*Log Cabin* or *Cary's*

Parmesan cheese—*Kraft Reduced Fat Parmesan Style Grated*

Reduced-fat cheese (shredded and sliced)—*Kraft 2% Reduced Fat*

Processed cheese—*Velveeta 2% Milk*

Shredded frozen potatoes—*Mr. Dell's* or *Ore Ida*

Reduced-fat peanut butter—*Peter Pan*, *Skippy*, or *Jif*

Spreadable fruit spread—*Welch's* or *Smucker's*

Chicken and beef broth—*Swanson*

Dry beef or chicken bouillon—*Wyler's Granules Instant Bouillon*

Tomato sauce—*Hunt's*

Canned soups—*Healthy Request*

Tomato juice—*Healthy Request*

Ketchup—*Heinz No Salt Added*

Pastrami and corned beef—*Carl Buddig Lean*

Luncheon meats—*Healthy Choice* or *Oscar Mayer*

Ham—*Dubuque 97% Fat Free* or *Healthy Choice*

Bacon bits—*Oscar Mayer* or *Hormel*

Kielbasa sausage and frankfurters—*Healthy Choice* or *Oscar Mayer Light*

Canned white chicken, packed in water—*Swanson*

Canned tuna, packed in water—*Starkist*

Canned salmon, packed in water—*Starkist*

95% to 97% lean ground sirloin beef or turkey breast

Crackers—*Nabisco Soda Fat Free* and *Ritz Reduced Fat*
Reduced-calorie bread (40 calories per slice)
Small hamburger buns (80 calories per bun)
Rice—instant, regular, and wild—*Minute Rice*
Instant potato flakes
Noodles, spaghetti, macaroni, and rotini pasta
Salsa
Pickle relish—dill, sweet, and hotdog
Mustard—Dijon, prepared yellow, and spicy
Unsweetened apple juice—*Musselman's*
Reduced-calorie cranberry juice cocktail—*Ocean Spray*
Unsweetened orange juice—*Simply Orange*
Unsweetened applesauce—*Musselman's*
Fruit—fresh, frozen, and canned in fruit juice
Vinegar—cider and distilled white
Lemon and lime juice (in small plastic fruit-shaped bottles,
   found in produce section)
Diet lemon-lime soda pop—*Diet Mountain Dew Caffeine Free*
Instant fruit beverage mixes—*Crystal Light*
Reduced-calorie chocolate syrup—*Hershey's Lite Syrup*
Sugar-free and fat-free ice cream—*Wells' Blue Bunny*

Remember, these are my suggestions. You are always free to use other national or local brands. Just keep in mind that if your choice is higher in fats and carbs, then you must adjust the recipe's nutritional data accordingly.

If you keep your pantry stocked with these products, you can whip up any recipe in this cookbook. I suggest you start a running list, and whenever you use up anything (or start to run low), remember to make a note of it. Your shopping trips will become quicker and thriftier!

Yes, But How Much Should It Be? A Healthy Exchanges Chopping Chart

Ever since I began sharing recipes all those years ago, readers have asked me to clarify what I mean by a particular size vegetable. They've also wanted to know if it was okay to use a little bit more of this or that in a specific recipe, rather than throw it away or freeze it.

I decided to provide you with a chart based on my experience preparing thousands of recipes over the years. I hope this will make it even easier to stir up Healthy Exchanges recipes each and every day. Now, everyone's idea of what a medium onion is might be slightly different. Some may think that it should chop up to ½ cup; others may believe that it produces at least a cup or even more. So to help you get a sense of a realistic "output" for my recipes, I've compiled the following chopping chart.

Just remember that in most cases we're talking about veggies with very minimal calorie counts. If your "medium" onion chops up to more than I suggest it should, you have my blessing to use it all. However, that does *not* mean that you can replace a small head of cabbage with a large one and expect the final quantity of the recipe to be the same!

Fruits

Apple:
    Medium = 1 cup chopped
Peach:
    Medium = ¾ cup chopped
Pear:
    Medium = 1 cup chopped

Vegetables

Broccoli:
    Small = 3 cups chopped
    Medium = 5 cups chopped
    Large = 7 cups chopped
Cabbage:
    Small = 4 cups chopped
    Medium = 6 cups chopped
    Large = 8 cups chopped
Carrots:
    Medium = ⅓ cup chopped
    Large = ⅔ cup chopped
Cauliflower:
    Small = 3 cups chopped
    Medium = 5 cups chopped
    Large = 7 cups chopped
Celery:
    Medium stalk = ⅓ cup chopped
Cucumber:
    Small = 1 cup chopped
    Medium = 2 cups chopped
Green or Red Bell Pepper:
    Small = ⅓ cup chopped
    Medium = ½ cup chopped
    Large = ¾ cup chopped

Lettuce:
   Small = 4 cups shredded
   Medium = 6 cups shredded
Onion:
   Small = ½ cup chopped
   Medium = ¾ cup chopped
   Large = 1 cup chopped
Potato:
   5-ounce raw = ¾ cup chopped
Tomato:
   Medium = ¾ cup chopped
   Large = 1 cup chopped
Turnips:
   Medium = ¾ cup chopped
Zucchini:
   Small = 1 cup chopped
   Medium = 2 cups chopped

JoAnna's Ten Commandments of Successful Cooking

A very important part of any journey is knowing where you are going and the best way to get there. If you plan and prepare before you start to cook, you should reach mealtime with foods to write home about!

1. **Read the entire recipe from start to finish** and be sure you understand the process involved. Check that you have all the equipment you will need *before* you begin.

2. **Check the ingredient list** and be sure you have *everything* and in the amounts required. Keep cooking sprays handy—while they're not listed as ingredients, I use them all the time (just a quick squirt!).

3. **Set out *all* the ingredients and equipment needed** to prepare the recipe on the counter near you *before* you start. Remember that old saying *A stitch in time saves nine*? It applies in the kitchen, too.

4. **Do as much advance preparation as possible** before actually cooking. Chop, cut, grate, or do whatever is needed to prepare the ingredients and have them ready before you start to mix. Turn the oven on at least ten minutes before putting food in to bake, to allow the oven to preheat to the proper temperature.

5. **Use a kitchen timer** to tell you when the cooking or baking time is up. Because stove temperatures vary slightly by manufacturer, you may want to set your timer for five minutes less than the suggested time just to prevent overcooking. Check the progress of your dish at that time, then decide if you need the additional minutes or not.

6. **Measure carefully.** Use glass measures for liquids and metal or plastic cups for dry ingredients. My recipes are based on standard measurements. Unless I tell you it's a scant or full cup, measure the cup level.

7. **For best results, follow the recipe instructions exactly.** Feel free to substitute ingredients that *don't tamper* with the basic chemistry of the recipe, but be sure to leave key ingredients alone. For example, you could substitute sugar-free instant chocolate pudding for sugar-free instant butterscotch pudding, but if you used a six-serving package when a four-serving package was listed in the ingredients, or you used instant when cook-and-serve is required, you won't get the right result.

8. **Clean up as you go.** It is much easier to wash a few items at a time than to face a whole counter of dirty dishes later. The same is true for spills on the counter or floor.

9. **Be careful about doubling or halving a recipe.** Though many recipes can be altered successfully to serve more or fewer people, *many cannot*. This is especially true when it comes to spices and liquids. If you try to double a recipe that calls for 1 teaspoon pumpkin-pie spice, for example, and you double the spice, you may end up with a too-spicy taste. I usually suggest increasing spices by 1½

times when doubling a recipe. If it tastes a little bland to you, you can increase the spice to 1¾ times the original amount the next time you prepare the dish. Remember: You can always add more, but you can't take it out after it's stirred in.

The same is true with liquid ingredients. If you wanted to **triple** a main dish recipe because you were planning to serve a crowd, you might think you should use three times as much of every ingredient. Don't, or you could end up with soup instead! If the original recipe calls for 1¾ cups tomato sauce, I'd suggest using 3½ cups when you **triple** the recipe (or 2¾ cups if you **double** it). You'll still have a good-tasting dish that won't run all over the plate.

10. **Write your reactions next to each recipe once you've served it.** Yes, that's right, I'm giving you permission to write in this book. It's yours, after all. Ask yourself: Did everyone like it? Did you have to add another half teaspoon of chili seasoning to please your family, who like to live on the spicier side of the street? You may even want to rate the recipe on a scale of 1☆ to 4☆, depending on what you thought of it. (Four stars would be the top rating—and I hope you'll feel that way about many of my recipes.) Jotting down your comments while they are fresh in your mind will help you personalize the recipe to your own taste the next time you prepare it.

The Recipes

How to Read a Healthy Exchanges Recipe

The Healthy Exchanges Nutritional Analysis

Before using these recipes, you may wish to consult your physician or health-care provider to be sure they are appropriate for you. The information in this book is not intended to take the place of any medical advice. It reflects my experiences, studies, research, and opinions regarding healthy eating.

Each recipe includes nutritional information calculated in three ways:

Healthy Exchanges Weight Loss Choices or Exchanges
Calories; Fat, Protein, Carbohydrates, and Fiber in grams;
   Sodium and Calcium in milligrams
Diabetic Exchanges
Carb Choices for those who prefer to count their carbs

In every Healthy Exchanges recipe, the Diabetic Exchanges have been calculated by a registered dietitian. All the other calculations were done by computer, using Food Processor II software.

When the ingredient listing gives more than one choice, the first ingredient listed is the one used in the recipe analysis. Due to inevitable variations in the ingredients you choose to use, the nutritional values should be considered approximate.

Please note the following symbols:

☆ This star means you should read the recipe's directions carefully for special instructions about **division** of ingredients.

❋ This symbol indicates **FREEZES WELL.**

Super-Duper

Soups and Stews

The very best soups and stews taste as if they have been bubbling away for hours, even days, and yet who really has that kind of time anymore? Over the years (and in my several dozen cookbooks) I've created lots of quick and delicious soup recipes; now, it gives me special pleasure to offer you some of my most satisfying and soul-stirring "potfuls" ever in this volume dedicated to the special talents of the pressure cooker. By compressing the time needed to tenderize meats and veggies, this miracle worker delivers old-fashioned flavors in a fraction of the time!

Let me tempt you with just a few of the special dishes I hope you'll place on your menu often: There's nothing more tummy-pleasing on a brisk fall evening than a bowl of my Creamy Chicken and Potato Soup, *brimming with chunks of meat and potatoes. Your family will never feel they're eating leftovers when you present them with rich and hearty* Tantalizing Turkey Vegetable Soup. *You're sure to please everyone from grandkids to great-grandparents with my cozy, old-fashioned* Fireside Beef Stew. *And you don't have to wait for a special occasion to win hearts and taste buds with* Cheesy Cauliflower and Ham Chowder!

Classic Chicken Rice Soup

The name says it all—the soul-satisfying, tummy-warming dish you've loved since you were a child! Why change what works—except to make it easier to prepare?   ☻   Serves 6 (1⅓ cups)

> 16 ounces skinned and boned uncooked chicken breast, cut
>   into bite-size pieces
> 2 (14-ounce) cans Swanson Lower Sodium Fat Free Chicken
>   Broth
> 1½ cups frozen cut carrots, thawed
> 1 cup diced celery
> ½ cup chopped onion
> ⅓ cup uncooked Minute Rice
> ¾ teaspoon poultry seasoning
> 1 teaspoon lemon pepper
> ¼ teaspoon black pepper

Spray a pressure cooker container with butter-flavored cooking spray. In prepared container, sauté chicken pieces for 5 minutes. Stir in chicken broth, carrots, celery, and onion. Add uncooked instant rice, poultry seasoning, lemon pepper, and black pepper. Mix well to combine. Place cover on cooker and bring to LOW pressure over medium heat. Lower heat to stabilize pressure and cook for 12 minutes. Remove from heat, wait for pressure to be released, remove cover, and stir. Let stand 5 to 10 minutes before serving.

HINT: Thaw carrots by rinsing in a colander under hot water for 1
    minute.

Each serving equals:

**171 Calories • 3 gm Fat • 26 gm Protein • 10 gm Carbohydrate • 393 mg Sodium •
45 mg Calcium • 2 gm Fiber**

DIABETIC EXCHANGES: 2 Meat • 1 Vegetable

CARB CHOICES: ½

Creamy Chicken Broccoli Noodle Soup

Instead of discovering the usual veggies in chicken noodle soup, invite your family to go for the gusto with this lusciously healthy combination. It's rich in nourishment and oh so tasty all at once!

Serves 4 (1¼ cups)

1 (14-ounce) can Swanson Lower Sodium Fat Free Chicken Broth
1½ cups diced cooked chicken breast
2 cups frozen chopped broccoli, thawed

1¼ cups uncooked noodles
1½ teaspoons lemon pepper
¼ teaspoon black pepper
1 (12-fluid-ounce) can Carnation Evaporated Fat Free Milk
3 tablespoons all-purpose flour

Spray a pressure cooker container with butter-flavored cooking spray. In prepared container, combine chicken broth, chicken, broccoli, and uncooked noodles. Add lemon pepper and black pepper. Mix well to combine. Place cover on cooker and bring to LOW pressure over medium heat. Lower heat to stabilize pressure and cook for 4 minutes. Remove from heat, wait for pressure to be released, remove cover, and stir. In a covered jar, combine evaporated milk and flour. Shake well to blend. Add milk mixture to soup mixture. Mix well to combine. Cook over medium heat for 4 to 5 minutes, stirring often.

HINTS: 1. If you don't have leftovers, purchase a chunk of cooked chicken breast from your local deli.
2. Thaw broccoli by rinsing in a colander under hot water for 1 minute.

Each serving equals:

255 Calories • 3 gm Fat • 28 gm Protein • 29 gm Carbohydrate • 513 mg Sodium • 304 mg Calcium • 3 gm Fiber

DIABETIC EXCHANGES: 2 Meat • 1 Fat-Free Milk • 1 Starch • 1 Vegetable

CARB CHOICES: 2

Chicken–Pea Soup Almondine

Looking for an elegant soup to launch your next dinner party, or just interested in treating yourself really well after a long day at work? Try a bowl of this sumptuous soup, which sparkles with a touch of added crunch. ☺ Serves 4 (1¼ cups)

> 1 (10¾-ounce) can Healthy Request Cream of Chicken Soup
> 1 cup water
> 1½ cups diced cooked chicken breast
> 1 cup frozen peas, thawed
> ¼ cup slivered almonds
> 1 teaspoon dried parsley flakes
> ¼ teaspoon black pepper
> 1 (12-fluid-ounce) can Carnation Evaporated Fat Free Milk

Spray a pressure cooker container with butter-flavored cooking spray. In prepared container, combine chicken soup and water. Add chicken, peas, almonds, parsley flakes, and black pepper. Mix well to combine. Place cover on cooker and bring to LOW pressure over medium heat. Lower heat to stabilize pressure and cook for 3 minutes. Remove from heat, wait for pressure to be released, remove cover, and stir. Stir in evaporated milk. Let set for 5 to 10 minutes before serving.

HINTS: 1. If you don't have leftovers, purchase a chunk of cooked chicken breast from your local deli.
2. Thaw peas by rinsing in a colander under hot water for 1 minute.

Each serving equals:

262 Calories • 6 gm Fat • 27 gm Protein • 25 gm Carbohydrate • 471 mg Sodium • 282 mg Calcium • 2 gm Fiber

DIABETIC EXCHANGES: 1½ Meat • 1 Fat-Free Milk • 1 Starch/Carbohydrate • 1 Fat

CARB CHOICES: 1½

Creamy Chicken and Potato Soup

This is what I might call a "Sunday dinner soup." Why? Because without sitting down to a time-consuming family meal, you can still enjoy a wonderfully meaty dish that is also chock-full of tender potatoes!   ☯   Serves 4 (1¼ cups)

> 1 cup chopped celery
> ½ cup chopped onion
> 2 cups diced cooked chicken breast
> 1½ cups diced raw potatoes
> 1 (10¾-ounce) can Healthy Request Cream of Chicken Soup
> 1 cup water
> 1½ teaspoons dried parsley flakes
> ¼ teaspoon black pepper
> 1 (12-fluid-ounce) can Carnation Evaporated Fat Free Milk

Spray a pressure cooker container with butter-flavored cooking spray. In prepared container, sauté celery and onion for 5 minutes. Stir in chicken and potatoes. Add chicken soup, water, parsley flakes, and black pepper. Mix well to combine. Place cover on cooker and bring to LOW pressure over medium heat. Lower heat to stabilize pressure and cook for 3 minutes. Remove from heat, wait for pressure to be released, and remove cover. Stir in evaporated milk. Let set for 5 to 10 minutes before serving.

HINT: If you don't have leftovers, purchase a chunk of cooked chicken breast from your local deli.

Each serving equals:

220 Calories • 4 gm Fat • 25 gm Protein • 21 gm Carbohydrate • 377 mg Sodium • 44 mg Calcium • 2 gm Fiber

---

DIABETIC EXCHANGES: 2½ Meat • 1 Starch/Carbohydrate • ½ Fat-Free Milk

---

CARB CHOICES: 1½

Farmhouse Chicken Pasta Soup

It's easy to imagine that this heartwarming soup came from an old-fashioned country farmhouse kitchen, where it bubbled for hours in a huge black kettle. But instead you stirred it up yourself, with one very smart appliance! ● Serves 4 (1½ cups)

> ½ cup chopped onion
> 1½ cups diced cooked chicken breast
> 2 (14-ounce) cans Swanson Lower Sodium Fat Free Chicken
>   Broth
> 1½ cups thinly sliced carrots
> 1½ cups thinly sliced celery
> ⅔ cup uncooked rotini pasta
> 1½ teaspoons dried parsley flakes
> 1 teaspoon lemon pepper
> ¼ teaspoon black pepper

Spray a pressure cooker container with butter-flavored cooking spray. In prepared container, sauté onion for 5 minutes. Add chicken and chicken broth. Mix well to combine. Stir in carrots, celery, uncooked rotini pasta, parsley flakes, lemon pepper, and black pepper. Place cover on cooker and bring to LOW pressure over medium heat. Lower heat to stabilize pressure and cook for 5 minutes. Remove from heat, wait for pressure to be released, remove cover, and stir. Let set for 5 to 10 minutes before serving.

HINT: If you don't have leftovers, purchase a chunk of cooked
    chicken breast from your local deli.

Each serving equals:

150 Calories • 2 gm Fat • 20 gm Protein • 13 gm Carbohydrate • 558 mg Sodium •
61 mg Calcium • 3 gm Fiber

DIABETIC EXCHANGES: 2 Meat • 1 Starch • 1 Vegetable

CARB CHOICES: 1

Pacific Chicken Chowder

Creamy, cheesy, and definitely breezy to fix—this scrumptious soup features a lavish blend of vegetables along with succulent chicken.

● Serves 4 (2 cups)

½ cup chopped onion
1½ cups diced cooked chicken breast
1 (15-ounce) can diced tomatoes, undrained
1½ cups frozen mixed vegetables, thawed
1 (10¾-ounce) can Healthy Request Cream of Mushroom
    Soup
1½ teaspoons dried parsley flakes
¼ teaspoon black pepper
1 (12-fluid-ounce) can Carnation Evaporated Fat Free Milk
¾ cup cubed Velveeta 2% Milk processed cheese

Spray a pressure cooker container with butter-flavored cooking spray. In prepared container, sauté onion for 5 minutes. Add chicken, undrained tomatoes, and mixed vegetables. Mix well to combine. Stir in mushroom soup, parsley flakes, and black pepper. Place cover on cooker and bring to LOW pressure over medium heat. Lower heat to stabilize pressure and cook for 3 minutes. Remove from heat, wait for pressure to be released, remove cover, and stir. Add evaporated milk and Velveeta cheese. Mix well to combine. Cook over medium heat for 4 to 5 minutes or until cheese melts, stirring often.

HINTS: 1. If you don't have leftovers, purchase a chunk of cooked chicken breast from your local deli.
2. Thaw mixed vegetables by rinsing in a colander under hot water for 1 minute.

Each serving equals:

302 Calories • 6 gm Fat • 29 gm Protein • 33 gm Carbohydrate • 939 mg Sodium •
465 mg Calcium • 4 gm Fiber

DIABETIC EXCHANGES: 3 Meat • 1 Fat-Milk Free • 1 Starch/Carbohydrate

CARB CHOICES: 2

Tantalizing Turkey
Vegetable Soup

The aroma beckons your loved ones to linger near the kitchen, but when you finally place this soup before them on the table, the applause begins! What a great way to use up leftover turkey—and what a good reason to plan for leftovers!

● Serves 4 (1½ cups)

> 1 (14-ounce) can Swanson Lower Sodium Fat Free Chicken Broth
> 1 (15-ounce) can diced tomatoes, undrained
> ¾ cup water
> 2 cups diced cooked turkey breast
> 1 cup chopped celery
> ½ cup chopped onion
> ½ cup chopped carrots
> ½ cup frozen cut green beans, thawed
> 2 teaspoons dried parsley flakes
> ¼ teaspoon black pepper

Spray a pressure cooker container with butter-flavored cooking spray. In prepared container, combine chicken broth, undrained tomatoes, and water. Add turkey, celery, onion, carrots, green beans, parsley flakes, and black pepper. Mix well to combine. Place cover on cooker and bring to LOW pressure over medium heat. Lower heat to stabilize pressure and cook for 8 minutes. Remove from heat, wait for pressure to be released, remove cover, and stir. Let set for 5 to 10 minutes before serving.

HINT: Thaw green beans by rinsing in a colander under hot water for 1 minute.

Each serving equals:

165 Calories • 1 gm Fat • 28 gm Protein • 11 gm Carbohydrate • 400 mg Sodium • 65 mg Calcium • 4 gm Fiber

DIABETIC EXCHANGES: 2½ Meat • 2 Vegetable

CARB CHOICES: 1

Simple Vegetable Beef Soup

This easy dish is great for those busy evenings when you want to feed your family well but you're all dashing off to one activity or another—soccer game, book club, you name it! Now you can race out the door fully satisfied. ☻ Serves 6 (¾ cup)

> 16 ounces extra-lean ground sirloin beef or turkey breast
> 1 cup reduced-sodium tomato juice
> 1 (14-ounce) can Swanson Lower Sodium Fat Free Beef
>   Broth
> 2 teaspoons Worcestershire sauce
> 1 (10-ounce) package frozen mixed vegetables, thawed
> 1 tablespoon fresh parsley or 1 teaspoon dried parsley flakes

Spray a pressure cooker container with butter-flavored cooking spray. In prepared container, brown meat. Add tomato juice, beef broth, Worcestershire sauce, mixed vegetables, and parsley. Mix well to combine. Place cover on cooker and bring to LOW pressure over medium heat. Lower heat to stabilize pressure and cook for 3 minutes. Remove from heat, wait for pressure to be released, remove cover, and stir. Let set for 5 to 10 minutes before serving.

HINT: Thaw mixed vegetables by rinsing in a colander under hot
    water for 1 minute.

Each serving equals:

127 Calories • 3 gm Fat • 17 gm Protein • 8 gm Carbohydrate • 295 mg Sodium •
18 mg Calcium • 2 gm Fiber

DIABETIC EXCHANGES: 2 Meat • ½ Starch

CARB CHOICES: ½

Country Hamburger Vegetable Soup

There's something so delicious about a soup pot simmering away with all kinds of delectable ingredients inside! With more than half a dozen veggies in this recipe, plus some hearty beef, you've got a winner. ☻ Serves 6 (1⅓ cups)

16 ounces extra-lean ground sirloin beef or turkey breast	1 tablespoon Worcestershire sauce
½ cup chopped onion	2 cups diced raw potatoes
1 (15-ounce) can diced tomatoes, undrained	1 cup thinly sliced carrots
	2 cups chopped cabbage
1 (10¾-ounce) can Healthy Request Tomato Soup	¾ cup frozen whole-kernel corn, thawed
	½ cup frozen peas, thawed
1½ cups water	1½ teaspoons dried parsley flakes

Spray a pressure cooker container with butter-flavored cooking spray. In prepared container, brown meat and onion for 5 minutes. Stir in undrained tomatoes, tomato soup, water, and Worcestershire sauce. Add potatoes, carrots, cabbage, corn, peas, and parsley flakes. Mix well to combine. Place cover on cooker and bring to LOW pressure over medium heat. Lower heat to stabilize pressure and cook for 5 minutes. Remove from heat, wait for pressure to be released, remove cover, and stir. Let set for 5 to 10 minutes before serving.

HINT: Thaw corn and peas by rinsing in a colander under hot water for 1 minute.

Each serving equals:

224 Calories • 4 gm Fat • 18 gm Protein • 29 gm Carbohydrate • 360 mg Sodium • 52 mg Calcium • 5 gm Fiber

DIABETIC EXCHANGES: 2 Meat • 1½ Vegetable • 1½ Starch/Carbohydrate

CARB CHOICES: 1½

Beefy Barley Vegetable Soup

I remember a funny story from a friend who wanted to make a barley soup but didn't quite understand how this hearty grain works. She poured a bunch of barley into her soup pot—and all the liquid immediately disappeared! You won't have that problem here because I've figured out exactly the right ratio of barley to liquid.

Serves 6 (1⅔ cups)

16 ounces extra-lean ground
    sirloin beef or turkey
    breast
1 (14-ounce) can Swanson
    Lower Sodium Fat Free
    Beef Broth
1 (10¾-ounce) can Healthy
    Request Tomato Soup
1 cup water
1 teaspoon Worcestershire
    sauce

1 (15-ounce) can diced
    tomatoes, undrained
1 cup diced celery
1 cup chopped onion
1 cup chopped carrots
1 cup finely chopped raw
    potatoes
1 cup frozen cut green beans,
    thawed
3 tablespoons barley
¼ teaspoon black pepper

Spray a pressure cooker container with butter-flavored cooking spray. In prepared container, brown meat. Add beef broth, tomato soup, water, and Worcestershire sauce. Mix well to combine. Stir in undrained tomatoes, celery, onion, carrots, potatoes, and green beans. Add barley and black pepper. Mix well to combine. Place cover on cooker and bring to LOW pressure over medium heat. Lower heat to stabilize pressure and cook for 15 minutes. Remove from heat, wait for pressure to be released, remove cover, and stir. Let set for 5 to 10 minutes before serving.

HINT: Thaw green beans by rinsing in a colander under hot water for 1 minute.

Each serving equals:

212 Calories • 4 gm Fat • 19 gm Protein • 25 gm Carbohydrate • 471 mg Sodium •
56 mg Calcium • 5 gm Fiber

DIABETIC EXCHANGES: 2 Meat • 2 Vegetable • 1 Starch

CARB CHOICES: 1

Momma Mia Minestrone

"Everything but the kitchen sink" goes into traditional Italian mine-strone, the truly fantastic vegetable soup that came to this country with all the immigrants who settled here. This soup is a feast in a bowl! ☻ Serves 4 (1¼ cups)

8 ounces extra-lean ground sirloin beef or turkey breast
½ cup chopped onion
½ cup shredded carrots
½ cup chopped celery
1 (14-ounce) can Swanson Lower Sodium Fat Free Beef
   Broth
1 (15-ounce) can diced tomatoes, undrained
2 tablespoons reduced-sodium ketchup
⅔ cup uncooked elbow macaroni
1½ teaspoons Italian seasoning
¼ teaspoon black pepper
¼ cup Kraft Reduced Fat Parmesan Style Grated Topping

Spray a pressure cooker container with olive oil–flavored cooking spray. In prepared container, sauté meat, onion, carrots, and celery for 5 minutes. Stir in beef broth and undrained toma-toes. Add ketchup, uncooked macaroni, Italian seasoning, and black pepper. Mix well to combine. Place cover on cooker and bring to LOW pressure over medium heat. Lower heat to stabilize pressure and cook for 5 minutes. Remove from heat, wait for pres-sure to be released, remove cover, and stir. When serving, top each bowl with 1 tablespoon Parmesan cheese.

Each serving equals:

212 Calories • 4 gm Fat • 16 gm Protein • 28 gm Carbohydrate • 511 mg Sodium • 84 mg Calcium • 3 gm Fiber

DIABETIC EXCHANGES: 2 Meat • 1½ Vegetable • 1 Starch

CARB CHOICES: 2

Grandma's Sausage and Corn Chowder

When I see "chowder" on a menu, I'm already imagining the thick, rich bowl that will soon be set before me. Each spoonful turns up new treasure—golden corn, yummy potatoes, the sizzle of "sausage," and so much more!   ☯   Serves 4 (1½ cups)

> 8 ounces extra-lean ground sirloin beef or turkey breast
> 1 cup chopped celery
> ½ cup chopped onion
> 1 (10¾-ounce) can Healthy Request Cream of Mushroom Soup
> 1 cup water
> ¾ cup diced cooked potatoes
> ¾ cup frozen whole-kernel corn, thawed
> 1½ teaspoons sage
> 1½ teaspoons dried parsley flakes
> ¼ teaspoon black pepper
> 1 (12-fluid-ounce) can Carnation Evaporated Fat Free Milk
> 3 tablespoons all-purpose flour

Spray a pressure cooker container with butter-flavored cooking spray. In prepared container, sauté meat, celery, and onion for 5 minutes. Stir in mushroom soup and water. Add potatoes, corn, sage, parsley flakes, and black pepper. Mix well to combine. Place cover on cooker and bring to LOW pressure over medium heat. Lower heat to stabilize pressure and cook for 5 minutes. Remove from heat, wait for pressure to be released, remove cover, and stir. In a covered jar, combine evaporated milk and flour. Shake well to blend. Add milk mixture to soup mixture. Mix well to combine. Cook over medium heat for 4 to 5 minutes, stirring often.

HINT: Thaw corn by rinsing in a colander under hot water for 1 minute.

Each serving equals:

268 Calories • 4 gm Fat • 20 gm Protein • 38 gm Carbohydrate • 467 mg Sodium • 328 mg Calcium • 2 gm Fiber

DIABETIC EXCHANGES: 1½ Meat • 1½ Starch/Carbohydrate • 1 Fat-Free Milk • ½ Vegetable

CARB CHOICES: 2½

Gringo Chili

We've got a glorious tradition in the United States when it comes to chili—why, we've all heard stories of cowboys dining on it during cattle drives out west. While its origin is South of the Border, it's a dish well-loved by everyone!   ☻   Serves 6 (1⅔ cups)

> 16 ounces extra-lean ground sirloin beef or turkey breast
> 1 cup chopped onion
> ½ cup chopped red bell pepper
> ½ cup chopped green bell pepper
> 1 (15-ounce) can diced tomatoes, undrained
> 1 (8-ounce) can Hunt's Tomato Sauce
> 2 cups reduced-sodium tomato juice
> 1 cup water
> 1 cup chunky salsa (mild, medium, or hot)
> 1 (15-ounce) can Bush's red kidney beans, rinsed and
>   drained
> 2 teaspoons chili seasoning
> 1 teaspoon dried parsley flakes
> ¼ teaspoon black pepper

Spray a pressure cooker container with butter-flavored cooking spray. In prepared container, brown meat, onion, red pepper, and green pepper for 5 minutes. Stir in undrained tomatoes, tomato sauce, tomato juice, water, and salsa. Add kidney beans, chili seasoning, parsley flakes, and black pepper. Mix well to combine. Place cover on cooker and bring to LOW pressure over medium heat. Lower heat to stabilize pressure and cook for 5 minutes. Remove from heat, wait for pressure to be released, remove cover, and stir.

Each serving equals:

203 Calories • 3 gm Fat • 19 gm Protein • 25 gm Carbohydrate • 750 mg Sodium • 60 mg Calcium • 5 gm Fiber

DIABETIC EXCHANGES: 2½ Meat • 2½ Vegetable • ½ Starch

CARB CHOICES: 1

Dilly Chili con Carne

I've always enjoyed creating recipes with a surprise ingredient or two, and this is one of my recent favorites. "There's something different about this chili," I said to my tasters. "See if you can figure out what it is." You know what? They did!

☉ Serves 6 (1⅓ cups)

> 16 ounces extra-lean ground sirloin beef or turkey breast
> 1½ cups chopped onion
> ½ cup chopped celery
> 2 cups reduced-sodium tomato juice
> ½ cup water
> 1 (8-ounce) can Hunt's Tomato Sauce
> 2 teaspoons Splenda Granular
> 2 teaspoons chili seasoning
> 1 tablespoon dill pickle juice
> 1 (15-ounce) can Bush's red kidney beans, rinsed and
>   drained

Spray a pressure cooker container with olive oil–flavored cooking spray. In prepared container, brown meat. Add onion, celery, tomato juice, water, tomato sauce, Splenda, chili seasoning, and dill pickle juice. Mix well to combine. Stir in kidney beans. Place cover on cooker and bring to LOW pressure over medium heat. Lower heat to stabilize pressure and cook for 10 minutes. Remove from heat, wait for pressure to be released, remove cover, and stir.

Each serving equals:

184 Calories • 4 gm Fat • 19 gm Protein • 18 gm Carbohydrate • 377 mg Sodium • 53 mg Calcium • 4 gm Fiber

DIABETIC EXCHANGES: 2½ Meat • 2 Vegetable • ½ Starch

CARB CHOICES: 1

Chunky Tex-Mex Chili

I've watched chili cook-offs on the Food Network, and I've been intrigued by the different contenders—some thinner, some thicker, some hotter, and some filled with unusual additions (alligator? buffalo?). This is a classic that you can eat with a fork!

● Serves 6 (1⅓ cups)

> 8 ounces extra-lean ground sirloin beef or turkey breast
> 1 cup coarsely chopped onion
> ½ cup coarsely chopped green bell pepper
> 1 (15-ounce) can diced tomatoes, undrained
> 2 cups reduced-sodium tomato juice
> 1 tablespoon Splenda Granular
> 1 (15-ounce) can Bush's red kidney beans, rinsed and
>   drained
> 1 cup frozen whole-kernel corn, thawed
> 2 teaspoons chili seasoning
> ¼ teaspoon black pepper

Spray a pressure cooker container with butter-flavored cooking spray. In prepared container, brown meat, onion, and green pepper for 5 minutes. Stir in undrained tomatoes, tomato juice, and Splenda. Add kidney beans, corn, chili seasoning, and black pepper. Mix well to combine. Place cover on cooker and bring to LOW pressure over medium heat. Lower heat to stabilize pressure and cook for 5 minutes. Remove from heat, wait for pressure to be released, remove cover, and stir.

HINT: Thaw corn by rinsing in a colander under hot water for 1
   minute.

Each serving equals:

162 Calories • 2 gm Fat • 12 gm Protein • 24 gm Carbohydrate • 185 mg Sodium •
56 mg Calcium • 5 gm Fiber

DIABETIC EXCHANGES: 1½ Meat • 1½ Vegetable • 1 Starch

CARB CHOICES: 1

Oriental Beef Stew

If America deserves to be called a melting pot—and I believe it is—then I expect to find the flavors of varied cultures holding hands in the same dish. Here's one that invites East and West to party together in your mouth! ◑ Serves 6 (⅔ cup)

> *16 ounces lean round steak, tenderized and cut into bite-size*
> *pieces*
> *¼ cup reduced-sodium soy sauce*
> *1 cup sliced onion*
> *1 cup sliced green bell pepper*
> *1½ cups sliced celery*
> *1 (2.5-ounce) jar sliced mushrooms, drained*
> *1 (8-ounce) can sliced water chestnuts, drained*
> *1 (10¾-ounce) can Healthy Request Cream of Mushroom*
> *Soup*
> *½ cup water*

Spray a pressure cooker container with butter-flavored cooking spray. In prepared container, brown steak pieces for 5 minutes. Stir in soy sauce, onion, green pepper, celery, mushrooms, and water chestnuts. Add mushroom soup and water. Mix well to combine. Place cover on cooker and bring to LOW pressure over medium heat. Lower heat to stabilize pressure and cook for 8 minutes. Remove from heat, wait for pressure to be released, remove cover, and stir.

HINT: Good served over rice.

Each serving equals:

205 Calories • 5 gm Fat • 26 gm Protein • 14 gm Carbohydrate • 523 mg Sodium • 70 mg Calcium • 3 gm Fiber

DIABETIC EXCHANGES: 2 Meat • 2 Vegetable

CARB CHOICES: 1

Fireside Beef Stew

Back in the 1940s, our great president Franklin Delano Roosevelt comforted the nation with his Fireside Chats on the radio. Now you can experience the same kind of comfort with a bowl of this mouthwatering supper dish.   ☁   Serves 6 (1 cup)

> 16 ounces lean round steak, tenderized and cut into bite-size
>   pieces
> 2 cups chopped carrots
> 1½ cups chopped celery
> 1 cup chopped onion
> 3 cups cubed unpeeled raw potatoes
> 1 cup water
> 1 (12-ounce) jar Heinz Fat Free Beef Gravy
> 1½ teaspoons dried parsley flakes
> ¼ teaspoon black pepper

Spray a pressure cooker container with butter-flavored cooking spray. In prepared container, brown steak pieces for 5 minutes. Stir in carrots, celery, onion, potatoes, and water. Add beef gravy, parsley flakes, and black pepper. Mix well to combine. Place cover on cooker and bring to LOW pressure over medium heat. Lower heat to stabilize pressure and cook for 15 minutes. Remove from heat, wait for pressure to be released, remove cover, and stir.

Each serving equals:

236 Calories • 4 gm Fat • 27 gm Protein • 23 gm Carbohydrate • 435 mg Sodium • 76 mg Calcium • 3 gm Fiber

DIABETIC EXCHANGES: 2 Meat • 1 Starch • 1 Vegetable

CARB CHOICES: 1

Dinnertime Stew

Living on a farm, you call your family to dinner any way you can, and since some may be far from the house when dinner's ready, you might use a big bell. Just as that clanging sound says "Dinnertime," so does the aroma of this stew!   ○   Serves 4 (1½ cups)

> *16 ounces lean round steak, tenderized and cut into bite-size*
> *   pieces*
> *1 cup chopped onion*
> *1½ cups coarsely chopped celery*
> *3 teaspoons Worcestershire sauce☆*
> *½ cup water*
> *1 teaspoon Wyler's Beef Granules Instant Bouillon*
> *1½ cups coarsely chopped carrots*
> *2 cups peeled and diced raw potatoes*
> *1 (8-ounce) can Hunt's Tomato Sauce*
> *2 teaspoons dried parsley flakes*
> *¼ teaspoon black pepper*

Spray a pressure cooker container with butter-flavored cooking spray. In prepared container, combine steak pieces, onion, celery, 1 teaspoon Worcestershire sauce, water, and bouillon. Cook for 5 minutes or until meat is browned. Add carrots and potatoes. Mix well to combine. Stir in tomato sauce, remaining 2 teaspoons Worcestershire sauce, parsley flakes, and black pepper. Place cover on cooker and bring to LOW pressure over medium heat. Lower heat to stabilize pressure and cook for 8 minutes. Remove from heat, wait for pressure to be released, remove cover, and stir.

Each serving equals:

268 Calories • 4 gm Fat • 30 gm Protein • 28 gm Carbohydrate • 481 mg Sodium • 70 mg Calcium • 5 gm Fiber

DIABETIC EXCHANGES: 3 Meat • 2 Vegetable • 1 Starch

CARB CHOICES: 1½

Quick Irish Stew

I finally got to visit the country called home by many of my beloved ancestors, and I've always enjoyed "connecting" with those ancestors by serving classic Irish dishes like this one. It's fast, it's filling, and it uses the bounty of the land. ● Serves 4 (1 cup)

> 16 ounces lean round steak, tenderized and cut into bite-size pieces
> 1½ cups chopped carrots
> 1½ cups chopped turnips
> 1½ cups chopped onion
> 2 cups diced unpeeled raw potatoes
> 1 (14-ounce) can Swanson Lower Sodium Fat Free Beef Broth
> 3 tablespoons all-purpose flour
> ¼ teaspoon black pepper

Spray a pressure cooker container with butter-flavored cooking spray. In prepared container, brown steak pieces for 5 minutes. Stir in carrots, turnips, onion, and potatoes. In a covered jar, combine beef broth, flour, and black pepper. Shake well to blend. Add broth mixture to beef mixture. Mix well to combine. Place cover on cooker and bring to LOW pressure over medium heat. Lower heat to stabilize pressure and cook for 12 minutes. Remove from heat, wait for pressure to be released, remove cover, and stir.

Each serving equals:

184 Calories • 4 gm Fat • 17 gm Protein • 20 gm Carbohydrate • 301 mg Sodium • 22 mg Calcium • 3 gm Fiber

DIABETIC EXCHANGES: 3 Meat • 2 Vegetable • 1 Starch

CARB CHOICES: 2

Speedy Savory Stew

Did you ever notice how quiet your dinner table becomes when people are enjoying what they're eating? Oh, there's definitely a few sounds—the "mmmm" of satisfaction, for one—but eating pushes conversation to the back burner! Serves 6 (1 cup)

16 ounces lean round steak, tenderized and cut into bite-size pieces
3 teaspoons Worcestershire sauce☆
½ cup chopped onion
1 cup chopped celery
1½ cups chopped carrots
3 cups diced raw potatoes
1 (10¾-ounce) can Healthy Request Tomato Soup
¼ cup water
1½ teaspoons dried parsley flakes
¼ teaspoon black pepper

Spray a pressure cooker container with butter-flavored cooking spray. In prepared container, brown steak pieces, 1 teaspoon Worcestershire sauce, onion, and celery for 5 minutes. Stir in carrots and potatoes. Add tomato soup, water, remaining 2 teaspoons Worcestershire sauce, parsley flakes, and black pepper. Mix well to combine. Place cover on cooker and bring to LOW pressure over medium heat. Lower heat to stabilize pressure and cook for 10 to 12 minutes. Remove from heat, wait for pressure to be released, remove cover, and stir.

Each serving equals:

200 Calories • 4 gm Fat • 17 gm Protein • 24 gm Carbohydrate • 243 mg Sodium • 37 mg Calcium • 3 gm Fiber

DIABETIC EXCHANGES: **2 Meat • 1 Starch • 1 Vegetable**

CARB CHOICES: **1½**

Nassau Pork Stew

This dish has a little of the tropics in it because I've used sweet potatoes in place of the classic Idaho, but the more intriguing switch is from beef to pork, a delectable meat that is less frequently used in stews and soups. I'd like to change that—what do you think? ☻ Serves 6 (¾ cup)

> 16 ounces lean pork tenderloin, cut into bite-size pieces
> 1½ cups diced raw sweet potatoes
> 1½ cups frozen cut green beans, thawed
> 1 cup chopped onion
> 2 cups frozen whole-kernel corn, thawed
> 1 (15-ounce) can diced tomatoes, undrained
> 1 cup reduced-sodium tomato juice
> 1½ cups water
> 2 tablespoons Splenda Granular
> 1½ teaspoons chili seasoning
> 1 teaspoon dried parsley flakes

Spray a pressure cooker container with butter-flavored cooking spray. In prepared container, brown pork pieces for 5 to 6 minutes. Add sweet potatoes, green beans, onion, and corn. Mix well to combine. Stir in undrained tomatoes, tomato juice, water, Splenda, chili seasoning, and parsley flakes. Place cover on cooker and bring to LOW pressure over medium heat. Lower heat to stabilize pressure and cook for 8 minutes. Remove from heat, wait for pressure to be released, remove cover, and stir.

HINT: Thaw green beans and corn by rinsing in a colander under hot water for 1 minute.

Each serving equals:

248 Calories • 4 gm Fat • 25 gm Protein • 28 gm Carbohydrate • 163 mg Sodium • 50 mg Calcium • 5 gm Fiber

DIABETIC EXCHANGES: 2 Meat • 2 Vegetable • 1 Starch

CARB CHOICES: 1½

Cheesy Cauliflower and Ham Chowder

Some foods just go together perfectly, and I think ham and cheese are a perfect pair, don't you? Here's the thing: I also believe that cauliflower and cheese are a dynamic duo—and so I blended all three together in this bountiful soup. ☺   Serves 6 (1⅓ cups)

3 cups fresh or frozen chopped
    cauliflower, thawed
1 (14-ounce) can Swanson
    Lower Sodium Fat Free
    Chicken Broth
½ cup chopped onion
1 cup chopped celery
1½ cups diced Dubuque 97%
    fat-free ham or any
    extra-lean ham

¼ teaspoon black pepper
1 (12-fluid-ounce) can
    Carnation Evaporated
    Fat Free Milk
3 tablespoons all-purpose flour
½ cup cubed Velveeta 2% Milk
    processed cheese

Spray a pressure cooker container with butter-flavored cooking spray. In prepared container, combine cauliflower, chicken broth, onion, and celery. Stir in ham and black pepper. Place cover on cooker and bring to LOW pressure over medium heat. Lower heat to stabilize pressure and cook for 5 minutes. Remove from heat, wait for pressure to be released, remove cover, and stir. In a covered jar, combine evaporated milk and flour. Shake well to blend. Add milk mixture and Velveeta cheese to cooker. Mix well to combine. Cook over medium heat for 4 to 5 minutes or until cheese melts, stirring often.

HINT: Thaw cauliflower by rinsing in a colander under hot water
    for 1 minute.

Each serving equals:

150 Calories • 2 gm Fat • 15 gm Protein • 18 gm Carbohydrate • 709 mg Sodium • 244 mg Calcium • 2 gm Fiber

DIABETIC EXCHANGES: 1½ Meat • 1 Fat-Free Milk • 1 Vegetable

CARB CHOICES: 1

Split Pea and Ham Soup

I've found that lots of men love split pea and ham soup, but they get to enjoy it too rarely because it takes time to prepare well. Here's where that glorious device the pressure cooker saves the day—and saves you so much time. ☻ Serves 4 (1½ cups)

> ½ cup dried split peas
> 4 cups water
> 1 cup diced Dubuque 97% fat-free ham or any extra-lean ham
> 1 cup peeled and chopped raw potatoes
> 1 cup chopped celery
> 1 cup grated carrots
> ½ cup chopped onion
> 1 teaspoon dried parsley flakes
> ¼ teaspoon black pepper
> ¼ cup Land O Lakes no-fat sour cream

Spray a pressure cooker container with butter-flavored cooking spray. In prepared container, combine peas and water. Add ham, potatoes, celery, carrots, and onion. Mix well to combine. Stir in parsley flakes and black pepper. Place cover on cooker and bring to LOW pressure over medium heat. Lower heat to stabilize pressure and cook for 14 minutes. Remove from heat, wait for pressure to be released, remove cover, and stir. When serving, top each bowl with 1 tablespoon sour cream.

Each serving equals:

173 Calories • 1 gm Fat • 11 gm Protein • 30 gm Carbohydrate • 240 mg Sodium • 67 mg Calcium • 8 gm Fiber

DIABETIC EXCHANGES: 1½ Meat • 1½ Starch • 1 Vegetable

CARB CHOICES: 1½

Creamed Ham and
Cabbage Chowder

Soup has always been the thrifty cook's way of making the food she (or he) has on hand go further. It's filling and flavorful, so your family feels well-fed, but it also allows you to turn leftovers into a lip-smacking supper. ☻ Serves 4 (2 cups)

> 1 (10¾-ounce) can Healthy Request Cream of Mushroom
>   Soup
> 1 cup water
> ½ cup chopped onion
> 1 cup chopped celery
> 1½ cups sliced carrots
> 2 cups diced raw potatoes
> 3 cups coarsely chopped cabbage
> 1½ cups diced Dubuque 97% fat-free ham or any extra-lean
>   ham
> 1½ teaspoons dried parsley flakes
> ¼ teaspoon black pepper
> ½ cup Land O Lakes Fat Free Half & Half

Spray a pressure cooker container with butter-flavored cooking spray. In prepared container, combine mushroom soup and water. Add onion, celery, carrots, potatoes, cabbage, and ham. Mix well to combine. Stir in parsley flakes and black pepper. Place cover on cooker and bring to LOW pressure over medium heat. Lower heat to stabilize pressure and cook for 5 minutes. Remove from heat, wait for pressure to be released, and remove cover. Stir in half & half. Let set for 5 to 10 minutes before serving.

Each serving equals:

229 Calories • 5 gm Fat • 15 gm Protein • 31 gm Carbohydrate • 614 mg Sodium • 127 mg Calcium • 4 gm Fiber

DIABETIC EXCHANGES: 2 Meat • 2 Vegetable • 1½ Starch/Carbohydrate

CARB CHOICES: 2

Southwest Corn and Ham Chowder

I've created so many corn chowder recipes over the years, and my husband, Cliff, has enjoyed every one. But he found this version especially appealing because it contains the spicy sizzle of the Southwest with the addition of salsa!

● Serves 4 (scant 1½ cups)

> 1 (10¾-ounce) can Healthy Request Cream of Mushroom Soup
> 1 cup water
> ½ cup chunky salsa (mild, medium, or hot)
> 1 teaspoon chili seasoning
> 1½ cups frozen whole-kernel corn, thawed
> 1 cup peeled and diced raw potatoes
> 1½ cups diced Dubuque 97% fat-free ham or any extra-lean ham
> ½ cup Land O Lakes Fat Free Half & Half

Spray a pressure cooker container with butter-flavored cooking spray. In prepared container, combine mushroom soup, water, salsa, and chili seasoning. Add corn, potatoes, and ham. Mix well to combine. Place cover on cooker and bring to LOW pressure over medium heat. Lower heat to stabilize pressure and cook for 5 minutes. Remove from heat, wait for pressure to be released, and remove cover. Stir in half & half. Let set for 5 to 10 minutes before serving.

HINT: Thaw corn by rinsing in a colander under hot water for 1 minute.

Each serving equals:

227 Calories • 3 gm Fat • 15 gm Protein • 35 gm Carbohydrate • 1,110 mg Sodium • 64 mg Calcium • 2 gm Fiber

DIABETIC EXCHANGES: 2 Meat • 2 Starch/Carbohydrate

CARB CHOICES: 2

Comforting Ham and Bean Soup

There's a reason kids love soup and sandwiches on cold, rainy days—it makes them feel "hugged" inside and out! Here's a terrific way to make sure they get their veggies at the same time!

● Serves 4 (1½ cups)

> ¾ cup shredded carrots
> ¾ cup chopped celery
> ½ cup chopped onion
> 1 cup diced Dubuque 97% fat-free ham or any extra-lean ham
> 2 (15-ounce) cans Bush's great northern beans, rinsed and drained
> 2½ cups water
> ¼ cup reduced-sodium ketchup
> 1½ teaspoons dried parsley flakes
> ¼ teaspoon black pepper

Spray a pressure cooker container with butter-flavored cooking spray. In prepared container, combine carrots, celery, onion, ham, and great northern beans. Add water, ketchup, parsley flakes, and black pepper. Mix well to combine. Place cover on cooker and bring to LOW pressure over medium heat. Lower heat to stabilize pressure and cook for 5 minutes. Remove from heat, wait for pressure to be released, remove cover, and stir. Let set for 5 to 10 minutes before serving.

Each serving equals:

189 Calories • 1 gm Fat • 13 gm Protein • 32 gm Carbohydrate • 205 mg Sodium • 75 mg Calcium • 10 gm Fiber

DIABETIC EXCHANGES: 2 Meat • 1½ Starch • 1 Vegetable

CARB CHOICES: 2

Ham and Bean Soup Pronto

Fast. Speedy. Quick. All those synonyms for getting you out of the kitchen in a flash—and this dish deserves every one! As long as you've got a few ingredients in the pantry, you're good to go!

● Serves 4 (2 full cups)

> 2 (15-ounce) cans Bush's great northern beans, rinsed and
>   drained
> 1½ cups diced Dubuque 97% fat-free ham or any extra-lean
>   ham
> 1 cup grated carrots
> 1 cup chopped celery
> ½ cup chopped onion
> 4 cups water
> ½ cup reduced-sodium ketchup
> 1 teaspoon dried parsley flakes
> ¼ teaspoon black pepper

Spray a pressure cooker container with butter-flavored cooking spray. In prepared container, combine great northern beans, ham, carrots, celery, onion, and water. Add ketchup, parsley flakes, and black pepper. Mix well to combine. Place cover on cooker and bring to LOW pressure over medium heat. Lower heat to stabilize pressure and cook for 5 minutes. Remove from heat, wait for pressure to be released, remove cover, and stir. Let set for 5 to 10 minutes before serving.

Each serving equals:

234 Calories • 2 gm Fat • 19 gm Protein • 35 gm Carbohydrate • 554 mg Sodium • 77 mg Calcium • 9 gm Fiber

DIABETIC EXCHANGES: 3 Meat • 2 Starch/Carbohydrate • 1 Vegetable

CARB CHOICES: 1½

Grandma's Stewed Bean Pot

Eating at Grandma's always promised to be a memorable experience, and it was even more so for me because one of mine ran a boardinghouse. This is her kind of dish, made super fast but no less tasty. ☻ Serves 6 (1⅓ cups)

> 3 (15-ounce) cans Bush's great northern beans, rinsed and
>   drained
> ½ cup finely chopped onion
> 1 cup frozen cut green beans, thawed
> 1 (15-ounce) can diced tomatoes, undrained
> ¼ cup reduced-sodium ketchup
> 2 cups water
> 2 cups diced Dubuque 97% fat-free ham or any extra-lean
>   ham
> 2 cups shredded cabbage
> ¼ teaspoon black pepper

Spray a pressure cooker container with butter-flavored cooking spray. In prepared container, combine great northern beans, onion, green beans, and undrained tomatoes. Add ketchup and water. Mix well to combine. Stir in ham, cabbage, and black pepper. Place cover on cooker and bring to LOW pressure over medium heat. Lower heat to stabilize pressure and cook for 5 minutes. Remove from heat, wait for pressure to be released, remove cover, and stir. Let set for 5 to 10 minutes before serving.

HINT: Thaw green beans by rinsing in a colander under hot water
    for 1 minute.

Each serving equals:

214 Calories • 2 gm Fat • 18 gm Protein • 31 gm Carbohydrate • 553 mg Sodium • 80 mg Calcium • 10 gm Fiber

DIABETIC EXCHANGES: 2½ Meat • 1½ Starch • 1 Vegetable

CARB CHOICES: 2

Heartland Hot Dog Chowder

I remember when we used to cater lunch at a local day care, and the little ones loved a cozy soup lunch, especially when it included another of their favorites: hot dogs, cut into tiny bits. Yum, yum!
● Serves 4 (1½ cups)

> 8 ounces Oscar Mayer or Healthy Choice reduced-fat
>   frankfurters, cut into bite-size pieces
> 1 cup chopped onion
> 1 cup chopped celery
> 1 (10¾-ounce) can Healthy Request Tomato Soup
> 1 (12-fluid-ounce) can Carnation Evaporated Fat Free Milk
> 1½ cups diced cooked potatoes
> ½ cup frozen whole-kernel corn, thawed
> 1½ teaspoons dried parsley flakes
> ¼ teaspoon black pepper

Spray a pressure cooker container with butter-flavored cooking spray. In prepared container, sauté frankfurter pieces, onion, and celery for 5 minutes. Stir in tomato soup and evaporated milk. Add potatoes, corn, parsley flakes, and black pepper. Mix well to combine. Place cover on cooker and bring to LOW pressure over medium heat. Lower heat to stabilize pressure and cook for 3 minutes. Remove from heat, wait for pressure to be released, remove cover, and stir. Let set for 5 to 10 minutes before serving.

HINT: Thaw corn by rinsing in a colander under hot water for 1 minute.

Each serving equals:

270 Calories • 2 gm Fat • 16 gm Protein • 47 gm Carbohydrate • 953 mg Sodium • 274 mg Calcium • 3 gm Fiber

DIABETIC EXCHANGES: 1½ Starch/Carbohydrate • 1 Fat-Free Milk • 1 Meat • 1 Vegetable

CARB CHOICES: 3

Tex-Mex Hot Dog Chili

Tangy, even spicy (depending on how much chili seasoning you choose to use), this new-style chili is a fun alternative to the traditional beef and beans recipe.   ○   Serves 4 (1½ cups)

> 8 ounces Oscar Mayer or Healthy Choice reduced-fat
>   frankfurters, cut into bite-size pieces
> ¾ cup chopped onion
> ¼ cup chopped green bell pepper
> 1 (15-ounce) can diced tomatoes, undrained
> 1 (10¾-ounce) can Healthy Request Tomato Soup
> 1 cup reduced-sodium tomato juice
> 1 cup frozen whole-kernel corn, thawed
> ⅔ cup uncooked elbow macaroni
> 2 teaspoons chili seasoning

Spray a pressure cooker container with butter-flavored cooking spray. In prepared container, sauté frankfurter pieces, onion, and green pepper for 5 minutes. Add undrained tomatoes, tomato soup, and tomato juice. Mix well to combine. Stir in corn, uncooked macaroni, and chili seasoning. Place cover on cooker and bring to LOW pressure over medium heat. Lower heat to stabilize pressure and cook for 3 minutes. Remove from heat, wait for pressure to be released, remove cover, and stir. Let set for 5 to 10 minutes before serving.

HINT: Thaw corn by rinsing in a colander under hot water for 1
    minute.

Each serving equals:

258 Calories • 2 gm Fat • 13 gm Protein • 47 gm Carbohydrate •
1,073 mg Sodium • 42 mg Calcium • 4 gm Fiber

DIABETIC EXCHANGES: 2 Starch/Carbohydrate • 2 Vegetable • 1 Meat

CARB CHOICES: 3

Hot Dog and Bean Soup

Dogs and beans are a classic combination on the plate, so I thought, why not stir them into my soup pot? Why not, indeed! The result is delicious! ☻ Serves 4 (1½ cups)

8 ounces Oscar Mayer or Healthy Choice reduced-fat
frankfurters, cut into bite-size pieces
1 cup chopped celery
1 cup shredded carrots
½ cup chopped onion
1 (10¾-ounce) can Healthy Request Tomato Soup
1 cup reduced-sodium tomato juice
1 cup water
1 (15-ounce) can Bush's great northern beans, rinsed and
drained
½ teaspoon Worcestershire sauce
1½ teaspoons dried parsley flakes
¼ teaspoon black pepper

Spray a pressure cooker container with butter-flavored cooking spray. In prepared container, sauté frankfurter pieces, celery, carrots, and onion for 5 minutes. Stir in tomato soup, tomato juice, and water. Add great northern beans, Worcestershire sauce, parsley flakes, and black pepper. Mix well to combine. Place cover on cooker and bring to LOW pressure over medium heat. Lower heat to stabilize pressure and cook for 3 minutes. Remove from heat, wait for pressure to be released, remove cover, and stir. Let set for 5 to 10 minutes before serving.

Each serving equals:

**202 Calories • 2 gm Fat • 13 gm Protein • 33 gm Carbohydrate •
1,196 mg Sodium • 64 mg Calcium • 6 gm Fiber**

DIABETIC EXCHANGES: 2 Meat • 1½ Starch/Carbohydrate • 1½ Vegetable

CARB CHOICES: 2

Creamy Tomato-Basil Soup

Basil is a remarkable herb, used dry or fresh. It brings out glorious flavors in any tomato-based dish, and it also transforms a dish made from a canned base into something spectacular!

Serves 4 (1½ cups)

½ cup diced onion
1 (10¾-ounce) can Healthy Request Tomato Soup
1 (15-ounce) can diced tomatoes, undrained
1 cup water
¾ cup uncooked noodles
1½ teaspoons dried basil leaves
¼ teaspoon black pepper
1 (12-fluid-ounce) can Carnation Evaporated Fat Free Milk

Spray a pressure cooker container with butter-flavored cooking spray. In prepared container, sauté onion for 5 minutes. Stir in tomato soup, undrained tomatoes, and water. Add uncooked noodles, basil, and black pepper. Mix well to combine. Place cover on cooker and bring to LOW pressure over medium heat. Lower heat to stabilize pressure and cook for 6 minutes. Remove from heat, wait for pressure to be released, remove cover, and stir. Stir in evaporated milk. Let set for 5 to 10 minutes before serving.

Each serving equals:

217 Calories • 1 gm Fat • 10 gm Protein • 42 gm Carbohydrate • 486 mg Sodium • 273 mg Calcium • 3 gm Fiber

DIABETIC EXCHANGES: 1½ Starch/Carbohydrate • 1 Fat-Free Milk

CARB CHOICES: 3

Green Bean and Noodle Tomato Soup

Tomato soup is a kid-pleasing favorite, but all children (and plenty of grown-ups, too) love novelty—something new and unexpected. I know how much Cliff loves green beans, so I decided to stir some into a velvety tomato soup—delish!   ☻   Serves 4 (1 cup)

> 1 (10¾-ounce) can Healthy Request Tomato Soup
> 1 cup reduced-sodium tomato juice
> 1 (15-ounce) can diced tomatoes, undrained
> 1 (15-ounce) can French-style green beans, rinsed and
>   drained
> ¾ cup uncooked noodles
> ½ teaspoon Worcestershire sauce
> ¼ teaspoon black pepper

Spray a pressure cooker container with butter-flavored cooking spray. In prepared container, combine tomato soup, tomato juice, and undrained tomatoes. Stir in green beans. Add uncooked noodles, Worcestershire sauce, and black pepper. Mix well to combine. Place cover on cooker and bring to LOW pressure over medium heat. Lower heat to stabilize pressure and cook for 3 minutes. Remove from heat, wait for pressure to be released, remove cover, and stir. Let set for 5 to 10 minutes before serving.

Each serving equals:

129 Calories • 1 gm Fat • 4 gm Protein • 26 gm Carbohydrate • 423 mg Sodium •
54 mg Calcium • 4 gm Fiber

DIABETIC EXCHANGES: 2½ Vegetable • 1 Starch/Carbohydrate

CARB CHOICES: 2

Neapolitan Tomato Bisque

Did you know that the word *Neapolitan* comes from the city of Naples, Italy? There are many different styles of cooking in Italy, often ranging from elegant and light to hearty and substantial. This luscious soup is somewhere in the middle.

○ Serves 4 (1½ cups)

> ½ cup chopped onion
> 1 (10¾-ounce) can Healthy Request Tomato Soup
> 1 (15-ounce) can diced tomatoes, undrained
> 1½ cups water
> ⅔ cup uncooked Minute Rice
> 1 teaspoon Italian seasoning
> ¼ cup Kraft Reduced Fat Parmesan Style Grated Topping
> 1 (12-fluid-ounce) can Carnation Evaporated Fat Free Milk
> 1 cup shredded fresh spinach leaves

Spray a pressure cooker container with olive oil–flavored cooking spray. In prepared container, sauté onion for 5 minutes. Stir in tomato soup, undrained tomatoes, and water. Add uncooked instant rice and Italian seasoning. Mix well to combine. Place cover on cooker and bring to LOW pressure over medium heat. Lower heat to stabilize pressure and cook for 3 minutes. Remove from heat, wait for pressure to be released, remove cover, and stir. Add Parmesan cheese, evaporated milk, and spinach. Mix well to combine. Serve at once.

Each serving equals:

229 Calories • 1 gm Fat • 10 gm Protein • 45 gm Carbohydrate • 605 mg Sodium • 280 mg Calcium • 3 gm Fiber

DIABETIC EXCHANGES: 1½ Starch/Carbohydrate • 1½ Vegetable • 1 Fat-Free Milk

CARB CHOICES: 3

Tom's Tomato Rice Soup

My son Tom is our webmaster for Healthy Exchanges (in addition to his regular job and the demands of being a busy father), and he doesn't have a lot of time to sit and linger over lunch. But I like knowing he's eating well, and this soup is both delicious and nutritious.   ☻   Serves 6 (1 cup)

1 cup finely chopped celery
½ cup finely chopped onion
1 (10¾-ounce) can Healthy Request Tomato Soup
1 (15-ounce) can diced tomatoes, undrained
2 cups water
¾ cup uncooked Minute Rice
2 teaspoons dried parsley flakes
¼ teaspoon salt
¼ teaspoon black pepper
½ cup Land O Lakes Fat Free Half & Half
⅓ cup Land O Lakes no-fat sour cream

Spray a pressure cooker container with butter-flavored cooking spray. In prepared container, sauté celery and onion for 5 minutes. Add tomato soup, undrained tomatoes, and water. Mix well to combine. Stir in uncooked instant rice, parsley flakes, salt, and black pepper. Place cover on cooker and bring to LOW pressure over medium heat. Lower heat to stabilize pressure and cook for 4 minutes. Remove from heat, wait for pressure to be released, remove cover, and stir. Stir in half & half and sour cream. Serve at once.

Each serving equals:

121 Calories • 1 gm Fat • 3 gm Protein • 25 gm Carbohydrate • 395 mg Sodium •
81 mg Calcium • 2 gm Fiber

DIABETIC EXCHANGES: 1 Starch/Carbohydrate • 1 Vegetable

CARB CHOICES: 1½

Tomato-Basil Rice Soup

Some people love a smooth soup, with nothing chunky or crunchy about it. My family has always preferred the kind that is filled with bits and pieces of veggies, meat, and noodles or rice. How about yours?

● Serves 4 (1 cup)

> ½ cup chopped onion
> 1 (10¾-ounce) can Healthy Request Tomato Soup
> 1 (15-ounce) can diced tomatoes, undrained
> 1 cup water
> ⅔ cup uncooked Minute Rice
> 1 teaspoon dried basil
> ¼ teaspoon black pepper
> ½ cup Land O Lakes Fat Free Half & Half

Spray a pressure cooker container with butter-flavored cooking spray. In prepared container, sauté onion for 5 minutes. Stir in tomato soup, undrained tomatoes, and water. Add uncooked instant rice, basil, and black pepper. Mix well to combine. Place cover on cooker and bring to LOW pressure over medium heat. Lower heat to stabilize pressure and cook for 3 minutes. Remove from heat, wait for pressure to be released, remove cover, and stir. Stir in half & half. Let set for 5 to 10 minutes before serving.

Each serving equals:

129 Calories • 1 gm Fat • 4 gm Protein • 26 gm Carbohydrate • 411 mg Sodium • 93 mg Calcium • 3 gm Fiber

DIABETIC EXCHANGES: 1½ Starch/Carbohydrate • 1 Vegetable

CARB CHOICES: 2

Creamy Italian Tomato Soup

Some people ask why I recommend the use of Italian seasoning instead of suggesting specific amounts of oregano, garlic, and so on. It's a good question, and I'd answer it by saying that I'm all for ease of preparation. I like knowing that the right proportions for the taste I want are already calculated for me.

● Serves 4 (1½ cups)

> ½ cup chopped onion
> 1 (10¾-ounce) can Healthy Request Tomato Soup
> 1 (15-ounce) can diced tomatoes, undrained
> ½ cup water
> 1 (2.5-ounce) jar sliced mushrooms, drained
> 1½ teaspoons Italian seasoning
> ¼ teaspoon black pepper
> 1 (12-fluid-ounce) can Carnation Evaporated Fat Free Milk
> 3 tablespoons all-purpose flour

Spray a pressure cooker container with olive oil–flavored cooking spray. In prepared container, sauté onion for 5 minutes. Add tomato soup, undrained tomatoes, water, mushrooms, Italian seasoning, and black pepper. Mix well to combine. Place cover on cooker and bring to LOW pressure over medium heat. Lower heat to stabilize pressure and cook for 3 minutes. Remove from heat, wait for pressure to be released, remove cover, and stir. In a covered jar, combine evaporated milk and flour. Shake well to blend. Add milk mixture to soup mixture. Mix well to combine. Cook over medium heat for 3 to 4 minutes, stirring often.

Each serving equals:

173 Calories • 1 gm Fat • 8 gm Protein • 33 gm Carbohydrate • 560 mg Sodium • 272 mg Calcium • 3 gm Fiber

DIABETIC EXCHANGES: 1½ Vegetable • 1 Fat-Free Milk • 1 Starch/Carbohydrate

CARB CHOICES: 2

Grandma's Homestyle Tomato-Rotini Soup

Sometimes I find myself standing in the pasta aisle, gazing at all the different shapes and thinking about recipes—which ones to use in which dish, which new ones to create a special dish for. I think rotini is perfect for this soup, but if your kids adore wagon wheels or *radiatore* (little radiators), go for it!   ☕   Serves 4 (1¼ cups)

> 1 tablespoon + 1 teaspoon I Can't Believe It's Not Butter!
>   Light Margarine
> ½ cup chopped onion
> 1 (15-ounce) can diced tomatoes, undrained
> 1 cup reduced-sodium tomato juice
> 2 tablespoons Splenda Granular
> 1½ teaspoons dried parsley flakes
> ¼ teaspoon black pepper
> ⅔ cup uncooked rotini pasta
> 1 (12-fluid-ounce) can Carnation Evaporated Fat Free Milk
> 3 tablespoons all-purpose flour

Spray a pressure cooker container with butter-flavored cooking spray. In prepared container, melt margarine. Stir in onion and sauté for 5 minutes. Add undrained tomatoes, tomato juice, Splenda, parsley flakes, and black pepper. Mix well to combine. Stir in uncooked rotini pasta. Place cover on cooker and bring to LOW pressure over medium heat. Lower heat to stabilize pressure and cook for 2 minutes. Remove from heat, wait for pressure to be released, remove cover, and stir. In a covered jar, combine evaporated milk and flour. Shake well to blend. Stir milk mixture into soup mixture. Cook over medium heat for 3 to 4 minutes, stirring often.

Each serving equals:

178 Calories • 2 gm Fat • 8 gm Protein • 32 gm Carbohydrate • 437 mg Sodium • 271 mg Calcium • 2 gm Fiber

DIABETIC EXCHANGES: 2 Vegetable • 1 Starch • ½ Fat-Free Milk • ½ Fat

CARB CHOICES: 2

Midwest Tomato Corn Soup

As they sing in "Oh, What a Beautiful Morning," the Midwest is definitely where the "corn is as high as an elephant's eye"—and so we stir corn into all kinds of recipes. Here, it adds sweetness and color, not to mention a bit of crunch, to this rosy soup.

Serves 4 (1¼ cups)

½ cup chopped onion
1 (10¾-ounce) can Healthy Request Tomato Soup
1 (15-ounce) can diced tomatoes, undrained
1 cup reduced-sodium tomato juice
1½ cups frozen whole-kernel corn, thawed
1 teaspoon dried basil
¼ teaspoon black pepper

Spray a pressure cooker container with butter-flavored cooking spray. In prepared container, sauté onion for 5 minutes. Stir in tomato soup, undrained tomatoes, and tomato juice. Add corn, basil, and black pepper. Mix well to combine. Place cover on cooker and bring to LOW pressure over medium heat. Lower heat to stabilize pressure and cook for 3 minutes. Remove from heat, wait for pressure to be released, remove cover, and stir. Let set for 5 to 10 minutes before serving.

HINT: Thaw corn by rinsing in a colander under hot water for 1
    minute.

Each serving equals:

149 Calories • 1 gm Fat • 4 gm Protein • 31 gm Carbohydrate • 471 mg Sodium •
36 mg Calcium • 4 gm Fiber

DIABETIC EXCHANGES: 2 Vegetable • 1 Starch

CARB CHOICES: 2

Zach's Italian Zucchini-Tomato Soup

Not everyone loves zucchini as much as my grandson Zach does, but anyone with a garden patch of zukes would be lucky to have someone like him to help use up the abundant crop!

● Serves 4 (1¼ cups)

> ½ cup chopped onion
> 1 (10¾-ounce) can Healthy Request Tomato Soup
> 1 (15-ounce) can diced tomatoes, undrained
> 2 cups water
> ⅔ cup uncooked Minute Rice
> 1 cup chopped unpeeled zucchini
> 1½ teaspoons Italian seasoning
> ¼ teaspoon black pepper
> ½ cup Land O Lakes Fat Free Half & Half
> ¼ cup Kraft Reduced Fat Parmesan Style Grated Topping

Spray a pressure cooker container with olive oil–flavored cooking spray. In prepared container, sauté onion for 5 minutes. Stir in tomato soup, undrained tomatoes, and water. Add uncooked instant rice, zucchini, Italian seasoning, and black pepper. Mix well to combine. Place cover on cooker and bring to LOW pressure over medium heat. Lower heat to stabilize pressure and cook for 15 minutes. Remove from heat, wait for pressure to be released, remove cover, and stir. Stir in half & half. When serving, top each bowl with 1 tablespoon Parmesan cheese.

Each serving equals:

177 Calories • 1 gm Fat • 5 gm Protein • 37 gm Carbohydrate • 512 mg Sodium • 85 mg Calcium • 3 gm Fiber

DIABETIC EXCHANGES: 1½ Starch/Carbohydrate • 1½ Vegetable

CARB CHOICES: 2½

Savory French Onion Soup

A pressure cooker is the ideal kitchen pal for making onion soup quickly, since the traditional version takes hours to produce that unique and intense onion flavor. ☻ Serves 4 (1 cup)

1 tablespoon + 1 teaspoon I Can't Believe It's Not Butter!
 Light Margarine
3 cups thinly sliced onion
1 (12-ounce) jar Heinz Fat Free Beef Gravy
2 cups water
1 teaspoon Worcestershire sauce
1½ teaspoons dried parsley flakes
¼ teaspoon black pepper
¼ cup Kraft Reduced Fat Parmesan Style Grated Topping
2 slices reduced-calorie white bread, toasted and cut into
 cubes
½ cup shredded Kraft reduced-fat mozzarella cheese

Spray a pressure cooker container with butter-flavored cooking spray. In prepared container, melt margarine. Stir in onion and sauté for 6 to 8 minutes or until tender. Add beef gravy, water, Worcestershire sauce, parsley flakes, and black pepper. Mix well to combine. Place cover on cooker and bring to LOW pressure over medium heat. Lower heat to stabilize pressure and cook for 3 minutes. Remove from heat, wait for pressure to be released, remove cover, and stir. Stir in Parmesan cheese. For each serving, place a quarter of the bread cubes in a soup bowl, spoon about 1 cup soup over bread cubes, and top with 2 tablespoons mozzarella cheese. Serve at once.

Each serving equals:

180 Calories • 4 gm Fat • 8 gm Protein • 28 gm Carbohydrate • 835 mg Sodium • 240 mg Calcium • 2 gm Fiber

DIABETIC EXCHANGES: 1½ Vegetable • 1 Starch/Carbohydrate • 1 Meat • ½ Fat

CARB CHOICES: 2

Ultra-Cheesy Veggie Soup

If you love cheese-based soups (and who doesn't?) but avoid them when you're dining out because you are concerned about calories, cholesterol, and fat, come home to a real delight! This super-duper celebration of cheese is good for you.

☻ Serves 4 (1¼ cups)

> 1 tablespoon + 1 teaspoon I Can't Believe It's Not Butter!
>   Light Margarine
> ½ cup chopped onion
> 3 cups frozen mixed vegetables, thawed
> 1 cup water
> 1 (12-fluid-ounce) can Carnation Evaporated Fat Free Milk
> 3 tablespoons all-purpose flour
> ¼ teaspoon black pepper
> 1 cup diced Velveeta 2% Milk processed cheese

Spray a pressure cooker container with butter-flavored cooking spray. In prepared container, melt margarine. Stir in onion and sauté for 5 minutes. Add mixed vegetables and water. Mix well to combine. In a covered jar, combine evaporated milk and flour. Shake well to blend. Stir milk mixture into vegetable mixture. Add black pepper. Mix well to combine. Place cover on cooker and bring to LOW pressure over medium heat. Lower heat to stabilize pressure and cook for 3 minutes. Remove from heat, wait for pressure to be released, remove cover, and stir. Add Velveeta cheese. Mix well to combine. Cook over medium heat for 4 to 5 minutes or until cheese melts, stirring often.

HINT: Thaw mixed vegetables by rinsing in a colander under hot water for 1 minute.

Each serving equals:

305 Calories • 5 gm Fat • 17 gm Protein • 48 gm Carbohydrate • 700 mg Sodium • 453 mg Calcium • 6 gm Fiber

DIABETIC EXCHANGES: 1½ Vegetable • 1 Meat • 1 Starch • 1 Fat-Free Milk • ½ Fat

CARB CHOICES: 3

Cream of Potato and Pea Soup

There are a number of ways to make a cream-style soup, but many of them produce a dish too high in fat to be enjoyed often. But when you stir some evaporated fat-free milk into your pot, you'll smile at the scrumptious result. ☺ Serves 4 (1 cup)

1 tablespoon + 1 teaspoon I Can't Believe It's Not Butter!
    Light Margarine
½ cup chopped onion
1 cup diced unpeeled raw potatoes
½ cup frozen peas, thawed
1¼ cups water
2 teaspoons dried parsley flakes
¼ teaspoon black pepper
⅔ cup instant potato flakes
1 (12-fluid-ounce) can Carnation Evaporated Fat Free Milk
¼ cup Land O Lakes no-fat sour cream
¼ cup Oscar Mayer or Hormel Real Bacon Bits

Spray a pressure cooker container with butter-flavored cooking spray. In prepared container, melt margarine. Stir in onion and sauté for 5 minutes. Add potatoes, peas, and water. Mix well to combine. Stir in parsley flakes and black pepper. Place cover on cooker and bring to LOW pressure over medium heat. Lower heat to stabilize pressure and cook for 3 minutes. Remove from heat, wait for pressure to be released, remove cover, and stir. Add instant potato flakes, evaporated milk, sour cream, and bacon bits. Mix well to combine. Cook over medium heat for 3 to 4 minutes, stirring often.

HINT: Thaw peas by rinsing in a colander under hot water for 1
    minute.

Each serving equals:

207 Calories • 3 gm Fat • 12 gm Protein • 33 gm Carbohydrate • 467 mg Sodium • 273 mg Calcium • 2 gm Fiber

DIABETIC EXCHANGES: 1 Fat-Free Milk • 1 Starch • ½ Meat • ½ Fat

CARB CHOICES: 2

Comforting Creamy Mushroom Soup

Okay, it would be nice to come home to a back rub or a magically clean house, but if neither of those prizes are available, why not treat yourself like a winner by fixing this marvelous mushroom dish? Its silky texture is irresistible! ☺ Serves 6 (1 cup)

> 2 tablespoons I Can't Believe It's Not Butter! Light
>   Margarine
> 6 cups chopped fresh mushrooms
> 1½ cups chopped onion
> ½ teaspoon dried minced garlic
> 1 cup water
> ¼ cup Land O Lakes Fat Free Half & Half
> 6 tablespoons Bisquick Heart Smart Baking Mix
> ¾ cup Land O Lakes no-fat sour cream
> 2 tablespoons chopped fresh parsley or 2 teaspoons dried
>   parsley flakes
> ¼ teaspoon black pepper

Spray a pressure cooker container with butter-flavored cooking spray. In prepared container, melt margarine. Stir in mushrooms, onion, and garlic. Sauté vegetables for 5 minutes, stirring often. In a large covered jar, combine water, half & half, and baking mix. Shake well to blend. Add milk mixture to mushroom mixture. Mix well to combine. Place cover on cooker and bring to LOW pressure over medium heat. Lower heat to stabilize pressure and cook for 3 minutes. Remove from heat, wait for pressure to be released, remove cover, and stir. Stir in sour cream, parsley, and black pepper. Serve at once.

Each serving equals:

123 Calories • 3 gm Fat • 5 gm Protein • 19 gm Carbohydrate • 189 mg Sodium • 79 mg Calcium • 1 gm Fiber

DIABETIC EXCHANGES: 1 Starch/Carbohydrate • 1 Vegetable • ½ Fat

CARB CHOICES: 1

Mexicali Cheese Soup

Here's a man-pleaser sure to win hearts at the height of football season! It's a truly savory dish that satisfies hungry fans—but the good news is that it also goes great with your favorite detective show.

● Serves 4 (scant 1 cup)

> 1 cup frozen whole-kernel corn, thawed
> ¾ cup diced cooked potatoes
> 1 cup chunky salsa (mild, medium, or hot)
> ¼ cup sliced ripe olives
> 1 cup water
> ¼ cup Land O Lakes Fat Free Half & Half
> 1½ cups cubed Velveeta 2% Milk processed cheese
> ¼ cup Land O Lakes no-fat sour cream
> ½ cup crushed Doritos Baked Corn Chips

Spray a pressure cooker container with olive oil–flavored cooking spray. In prepared container, combine corn, potatoes, salsa, and olives. Add water and half & half. Mix well to combine. Place cover on cooker and bring to LOW pressure over medium heat. Lower heat to stabilize pressure and cook for 3 minutes. Remove from heat, wait for pressure to be released, remove cover, and stir. Add Velveeta cheese. Mix well to combine. Cook over medium heat for 4 to 5 minutes or until cheese melts, stirring often. When serving, top each bowl with 1 tablespoon sour cream and 2 tablespoons crushed corn chips.

HINT: Thaw corn by rinsing in a colander under hot water for 1 minute.

Each serving equals:

269 Calories • 9 gm Fat • 11 gm Protein • 36 gm Carbohydrate •
1,246 mg Sodium • 308 mg Calcium • 4 gm Fiber

DIABETIC EXCHANGES: 2 Starch/Carbohydrate • 1½ Meat • ½ Vegetable

CARB CHOICES: 2½

Corny Corn Chowder

I remember a song lyric that reminded us that "too much is not enough," and this soup illustrates that perfectly! I've mixed in corn kernels and creamed corn to deepen and enrich the flavor and texture, and it's *just* enough. ☻ Serves 6 (1⅓ cups)

2 tablespoons I Can't Believe
    It's Not Butter! Light
    Margarine
1 cup chopped onion
2½ cups frozen whole-kernel
    corn, thawed
1 (8-ounce) can cream-style
    corn
½ cup diced raw potatoes

1 (15-ounce) can diced
    tomatoes, undrained
1½ cups water☆
2 tablespoons cornstarch
1 (12-fluid-ounce) can
    Carnation Evaporated
    Fat Free Milk
6 tablespoons chopped fresh
    parsley

Spray a pressure cooker container with butter-flavored cooking spray. In prepared container, melt margarine. Stir in onion and sauté for 5 minutes. Add whole-kernel corn, cream-style corn, potatoes, undrained tomatoes, and ½ cup water. Mix well to combine. Cook over medium heat for 3 minutes. In a small bowl, combine ¼ cup water and cornstarch using a wire whisk. Add cornstarch mixture and remaining ¾ cup water to corn mixture. Mix well to combine. Place cover on cooker and bring to LOW pressure over medium heat. Lower heat to stabilize pressure and cook for 3 minutes. Remove from heat, wait for pressure to be released, remove cover, and stir. Add evaporated milk. Mix well to combine. Let set for 5 to 10 minutes. When serving, sprinkle 1 tablespoon parsley over top of each bowl.

HINT: Thaw corn by rinsing in a colander under hot water for 1 minute.

Each serving equals:

206 Calories • 2 gm Fat • 7 gm Protein • 40 gm Carbohydrate • 223 mg Sodium • 192 mg Calcium • 3 gm Fiber

DIABETIC EXCHANGES: 1½ Starch • 1 Vegetable • ½ Fat-Free Milk • ½ Fat

CARB CHOICES: 2½

Cheesy Corn Chowder

If your kids can't get enough cheese, here's a dish to win big smiles from them. It's a great fall or winter lunch soup, nutritious and delicious—especially when served with a favorite sandwich.

◐ Serves 4 (1¼ cups)

> ½ cup chopped onion
> 1 (10¾-ounce) can Healthy Request Cream of Mushroom
>   Soup
> ¾ cup water
> 1 (8-ounce) can cream-style corn
> ¾ cup diced cooked potatoes
> ½ cup frozen whole-kernel corn, thawed
> 1½ teaspoons dried parsley flakes
> ¼ teaspoon black pepper
> 1 (12-fluid-ounce) can Carnation Evaporated Fat Free Milk
> 1 cup cubed Velveeta 2% Milk processed cheese

Spray a pressure cooker container with butter-flavored cooking spray. In prepared container, sauté onion for 5 minutes. Add mushroom soup, water, and cream-style corn. Mix well to combine. Stir in potatoes, whole-kernel corn, parsley flakes, and black pepper. Place cover on cooker and bring to LOW pressure over medium heat. Lower heat to stabilize pressure and cook for 3 minutes. Remove from heat, wait for pressure to be released, remove cover, and stir. Add evaporated milk and Velveeta cheese. Mix well to combine. Cook over medium heat for 4 to 5 minutes or until cheese melts, stirring often.

HINT: Thaw whole-kernel corn by rinsing in a colander under hot water for 1 minute.

Each serving equals:

277 Calories • 5 gm Fat • 14 gm Protein • 44 gm Carbohydrate • 861 mg Sodium • 475 mg Calcium • 2 gm Fiber

DIABETIC EXCHANGES: 1½ Starch/Carbohydrate • 1 Fat-Free Milk • 1 Meat

CARB CHOICES: 3

Cheesy Tater Chowder

You could make this chowder with any potato, but using red potatoes provides great color, good texture, and lots of vitamins, too! What a delightful duet—potatoes and cheese.

Serves 4 (1½ cups)

> 2 cups diced unpeeled raw red potatoes
> 1 cup shredded carrots
> 1 cup chopped celery
> ½ cup chopped onion
> 1½ cups water
> 1 tablespoon dried parsley flakes
> 1 tablespoon Worcestershire sauce
> ¼ teaspoon black pepper
> 1 (12-fluid-ounce) can Carnation Evaporated Fat Free Milk
> 3 tablespoons all-purpose flour
> 1½ cups cubed Velveeta 2% Milk processed cheese

Spray a pressure cooker container with butter-flavored cooking spray. In prepared container, combine potatoes, carrots, celery, onion, and water. Add parsley flakes, Worcestershire sauce, and black pepper. Mix well to combine. Place cover on cooker and bring to LOW pressure over medium heat. Lower heat to stabilize pressure and cook for 4 minutes. Remove from heat, wait for pressure to be released, remove cover, and stir. In a covered jar, combine evaporated milk and flour. Shake well to blend. Add milk mixture and Velveeta cheese to cooker. Mix well to combine. Cook over medium heat for 4 to 5 minutes or until cheese melts, stirring often.

Each serving equals:

273 Calories • 5 gm Fat • 17 gm Protein • 40 gm Carbohydrate • 888 mg Sodium • 526 mg Calcium • 3 gm Fiber

DIABETIC EXCHANGES: 1½ Meat • 1 Starch/Carbohydrate • 1 Fat-Free Milk • 1 Vegetable

CARB CHOICES: 2½

Broccoli Chowder

Frozen broccoli is such a useful cooking ingredient. I always watch for sales and keep plenty on hand. In this dish, it provides color and crunch in every bite.   ○   Serves 4 (1¼ cups)

½ cup chopped onion
1 cup peeled and diced raw potatoes
2 cups frozen cut broccoli, thawed
1 cup frozen whole-kernel corn, thawed
½ teaspoon lemon pepper
1 (10¾-ounce) can Healthy Request Cream of Celery Soup
1 teaspoon Wyler's Chicken Granules Instant Bouillon
1 cup water

Spray a pressure cooker container with butter-flavored cooking spray. In prepared container, sauté onion for 5 minutes. Add potatoes, broccoli, corn, and lemon pepper. Mix well to combine. Stir in celery soup, dry chicken bouillon, and water. Place cover on cooker and bring to LOW pressure over medium heat. Lower heat to stabilize pressure and cook for 5 minutes. Remove from heat, wait for pressure to be released, remove cover, and stir. Let set for 5 to 10 minutes before serving.

HINT: Thaw broccoli and corn by rinsing in a colander under hot water for 1 minute.

Each serving equals:

160 Calories • 4 gm Fat • 5 gm Protein • 26 gm Carbohydrate • 670 mg Sodium • 79 mg Calcium • 4 gm Fiber

DIABETIC EXCHANGES: 1½ Starch/Carbohydrate • 1 Vegetable

CARB CHOICES: 1½

Under the Sea Tuna Chowder

Tuna is such a thrifty protein source, it can be a great choice for lunch or dinner when you've got a hungry family to feed. This hearty soup is both inexpensive and fast.

● Serves 4 (1¼ cups)

¾ cup diced celery
¼ cup chopped onion
1 (10¾-ounce) can Healthy Request Cream of Mushroom or
*   Cream of Celery Soup*
1 cup water
1 (6-ounce) can white tuna, packed in water, drained and
*   flaked*
1½ cups diced cooked potatoes
½ cup frozen peas, thawed
1 (2-ounce) jar sliced pimiento, drained
1 teaspoon dried parsley flakes
¼ teaspoon black pepper
½ cup Land O Lakes Fat Free Half & Half

Spray a pressure cooker container with butter-flavored cooking spray. In prepared container, sauté celery and onion for 5 minutes. Stir in soup and water. Add tuna, potatoes, peas, pimiento, parsley flakes, and black pepper. Mix well to combine. Place cover on cooker and bring to LOW pressure over medium heat. Lower heat to stabilize pressure and cook for 3 minutes. Remove from heat, wait for pressure to be released, remove cover, and stir. Stir in half & half. Let set for 5 to 10 minutes before serving.

HINT: Thaw peas by rinsing in a colander under hot water for 1 minute.

Each serving equals:

184 Calories • 4 gm Fat • 14 gm Protein • 23 gm Carbohydrate • 248 mg Sodium • 88 mg Calcium • 2 gm Fiber

DIABETIC EXCHANGES: 1½ Meat • 1½ Starch/Carbohydrate

CARB CHOICES: 1½

Splendid Sides and Veggies

Sometimes I feel that calling these scrumptious dishes "sides" makes it seem as if they don't deserve the same attention the entrée gets. And yet nutritionists encourage us to fill our plates with more veggies than meat for better and more balanced health. So, these "secondary" dishes actually take up more room in our stomachs and on our tables. Hmm—I'm glad I've given these "featured players" lots of attention in this cookbook. They may not grab the spotlight, but they deserve plenty of applause!

You'll feel as if there's a party going on when you serve yourself some Majestic Mashed Potatoes—*they're a treat worthy of your most honored guests, but never forget to treat yourself like company, too! Your tomato patch will be oh-so-proud when you fix* Homemade Stewed Tomatoes *and revel in their straight-from-the-sun sweetness. Nothing says New England like a classic vegetable dish such as* Boston Bean Pot—*hearty and filling in every way. And you don't have to stand on your head or dance a jig to enjoy my* Nutty Green Beans—*but feel free to do so if it makes you feel good!*

Asparagus in Dijon Butter

If you find yourself with a gorgeous bunch of fresh asparagus picked up from a farm stand but you're not sure what to do with it, here's the recipe for you! The pressure cooker helps flavor this delicate veggie beautifully. ◐ Serves 4 (½ cup)

> 3 cups fresh or frozen chopped asparagus, thawed
> 2 tablespoons water
> 1 tablespoon Grey Poupon Country Style Dijon Mustard
> 2 tablespoons I Can't Believe It's Not Butter! Light
>   Margarine
> ¼ teaspoon black pepper

Spray a pressure cooker container with butter-flavored cooking spray. In prepared container, combine asparagus, water, mustard, margarine, and black pepper. Place cover on cooker and bring to LOW pressure over medium heat. Lower heat to stabilize pressure and cook for 6 minutes. Remove from heat, wait for pressure to be released, remove cover, and stir.

HINT: Thaw asparagus by rinsing in a colander under hot water for
    1 minute.

Each serving equals:

**42 Calories • 2 gm Fat • 2 gm Protein • 4 gm Carbohydrate • 160 mg Sodium •
25 mg Calcium • 2 gm Fiber**

DIABETIC EXCHANGES: 1½ Vegetable • ½ Fat

CARB CHOICES: 0

Old-Time Harvard Beets

One of the oldest universities in America, Harvard is known for the brainy students it attracts—and also for its school color, crimson. This dish takes raw beets and transforms them into something spectacular.   ☻   Serves 4 (¾ cup)

3 cups peeled and sliced raw beets
½ cup hot water
¼ cup cold water
¼ cup white distilled vinegar
1 tablespoon cornstarch
½ cup Splenda Granular
2 tablespoons I Can't Believe It's Not Butter! Light
    Margarine
¼ teaspoon table salt

In a pressure cooker container, combine beets and hot water. Place cover on cooker and bring to HIGH pressure over medium heat. Lower heat to stabilize pressure and cook for 10 minutes. Remove from heat, wait for pressure to be released, and remove cover. Drain, reserving ¼ cup liquid, and return beets to pressure cooker container. In a covered jar, combine cold water, vinegar, and cornstarch. Shake well to blend. Pour mixture into container with beets. Mix well to combine. Stir in reserved beet liquid, Splenda, margarine, and salt. Cook over medium-low heat for 2 minutes or until mixture thickens, stirring often.

Each serving equals:

**87 Calories • 3 gm Fat • 1 gm Protein • 14 gm Carbohydrate • 294 mg Sodium •
18 mg Calcium • 2 gm Fiber**

DIABETIC EXCHANGES: 1½ Vegetable • ½ Fat

CARB CHOICES: 1

Cheesy Broccoli

Luscious and nutritious, all at once? I proved beyond a doubt that it's possible when I fixed this grand combo of crunchy vegetable and creamy cheese. ☺ Serves 6 (¾ cup)

> 4 cups fresh or frozen chopped broccoli, thawed
> ½ cup chopped onion
> ½ cup water
> 1 (10¾-ounce) can Healthy Request Cream of Mushroom
>   Soup
> 2 tablespoons Land O Lakes Fat Free Half & Half
> ½ teaspoon Worcestershire sauce
> ¾ cup cubed Velveeta 2% Milk processed cheese
> 2 tablespoons I Can't Believe It's Not Butter! Light
>   Margarine
> ¼ teaspoon black pepper

In a pressure cooker container, combine broccoli, onion, and water. Place cover on cooker and bring to LOW pressure over medium heat. Lower heat to stabilize pressure and cook for 6 minutes. Remove from heat, wait for pressure to be released, and remove cover. Drain and return broccoli mixture to pressure cooker container. Add mushroom soup, half & half, and Worcestershire sauce. Mix well to combine. Stir in Velveeta cheese, margarine, and black pepper. Cook over medium heat for 2 to 3 minutes or until cheese melts, stirring often.

HINT: Thaw broccoli by rinsing in a colander under hot water for 1 minute.

Each serving equals:

100 Calories • 4 gm Fat • 5 gm Protein • 11 gm Carbohydrate • 497 mg Sodium • 160 mg Calcium • 1 gm Fiber

DIABETIC EXCHANGES: 1½ Vegetable • ½ Meat • ½ Starch/Carbohydrate

CARB CHOICES: 1

Broccoli-Cauliflower-Carrot Medley

Have you been a little disappointed with the taste result when cooking a bag of frozen veggies on your stovetop? Maybe they turned out a bit watery or less than full of flavor? Preparing them in your cooker will change all that once and for all!

○ Serves 4 (1 cup)

> 2 cups fresh coarsely chopped broccoli
> 1½ cups fresh or frozen chopped cauliflower, thawed
> 1 cup fresh or frozen sliced carrots, thawed
> ½ cup water
> 1 tablespoon + 1 teaspoon I Can't Believe It's Not Butter!
>   Light Margarine
> 1 teaspoon lemon pepper

In a pressure cooker container, combine broccoli, cauliflower, carrots, and water. Place cover on cooker and bring to LOW pressure over medium heat. Lower heat to stabilize pressure and cook for 3 minutes. Remove from heat, wait for pressure to be released, and remove cover. Drain and return vegetables to pressure cooker container. Add margarine and lemon pepper. Mix well to combine. Serve at once.

HINT: Thaw cauliflower and carrots by rinsing in a colander under hot water for 1 minute.

Each serving equals:

54 Calories • 2 gm Fat • 2 gm Protein • 7 gm Carbohydrate • 199 mg Sodium • 37 mg Calcium • 2 gm Fiber

DIABETIC EXCHANGES: 2 Vegetable • ½ Fat

CARB CHOICES: ½

Cauliflower in Mustard Sauce

If you're a fan of the "cruciferous" vegetables, the ones that take the longest to cook, then you already know that pressure cooking is the way to go! They're ready so quickly—and they brim with flavor.

☻ Serves 4 (½ cup)

3 cups raw cauliflower
½ cup water
1 teaspoon prepared yellow mustard
¼ teaspoon dried parsley flakes
⅛ teaspoon paprika
3 tablespoons I Can't Believe It's Not Butter! Light
*   Margarine, melted*

Spray a pressure cooker container with butter-flavored cooking spray. In prepared container, place cauliflower and water. Place cover on cooker and bring to LOW pressure over medium heat. Lower heat to stabilize pressure and cook for 3 minutes. Remove from heat, wait for pressure to be released, and remove cover. Drain and return cauliflower to pressure cooker container. In a small bowl, combine mustard, parsley flakes, paprika, and melted margarine. Spread mixture over cauliflower. Cook over low heat, for 3 to 4 minutes until hot, stirring occasionally.

Each serving equals:

**56 Calories • 4 gm Fat • 1 gm Protein • 4 gm Carbohydrate • 139 mg Sodium •
18 mg Calcium • 2 gm Fiber**

DIABETIC EXCHANGES: 1 Fat • 1 Vegetable

CARB CHOICES: 0

Cheesy Cabbage

Cabbage has so much healthy fiber, it's great for your body—but did you ever think of serving it with a scrumptious cheese sauce? This sensational side dish is appealing to young and old.

○ Serves 4 (¾ cup)

> 6 cups shredded cabbage
> ½ cup water
> ½ cup Land O Lakes Fat Free Half & Half
> 3 tablespoons all-purpose flour
> ¾ cup cubed Velveeta 2% Milk processed cheese
> ¼ teaspoon black pepper
> 1 tablespoon + 1 teaspoon I Can't Believe It's Not Butter!
>   Light Margarine

In a pressure cooker container, combine cabbage and water. Place cover on cooker and bring to HIGH pressure over medium heat. Lower heat to stabilize pressure and cook for 3 minutes. Remove from heat, wait for pressure to be released, and remove cover. Drain and return cabbage to pressure cooker container. In a covered jar, combine half & half and flour. Shake well to blend. Pour milk mixture over cabbage. Add Velveeta cheese and black pepper. Mix well to combine. Cook over medium-low heat for 2 minutes or until sauce thickens and cheese melts, stirring often. Just before serving, stir in margarine.

Each serving equals:

124 Calories • 4 gm Fat • 7 gm Protein • 15 gm Carbohydrate • 431 mg Sodium • 221 mg Calcium • 2 gm Fiber

DIABETIC EXCHANGES: 1 Meat • 1 Vegetable • ½ Starch

CARB CHOICES: 1

Easy "Fried" Cabbage

I had to put "fried" in quotation marks because there's not a drop of oil in sight, only a little light margarine—but oh, the cooking magic that occurs when you do it "under pressure." This is a real savory surprise. ☺ Serves 4 (½ cup)

> 2 tablespoons I Can't Believe It's Not Butter! Light Margarine
> 4 cups coarsely cut cabbage
> ½ teaspoon table salt

Spray a pressure cooker container with butter-flavored cooking spray. In prepared container, melt margarine. Stir in cabbage and salt. Place cover on cooker and bring to LOW pressure over medium heat. Lower heat to stabilize pressure and cook for 5 minutes. Remove from heat, wait for pressure to be released, remove cover, and stir.

Each serving equals:

38 Calories • 2 gm Fat • 1 gm Protein • 4 gm Carbohydrate • 371 mg Sodium • 34 mg Calcium • 1 gm Fiber

DIABETIC EXCHANGES: ½ Fat • 1 Free Food

CARB CHOICES: 0

Tangy Red Cabbage

My ancestors from eastern Europe loved cooking red cabbage with a sweet and tangy zing to it, but getting it right took a long while on the stovetop. Now you can enjoy those old-fashioned flavors a whole lot faster! ◐ Serves 4 (¾ cup)

> 4 cups shredded red cabbage
> 1 cup (1 medium) cored, peeled, and chopped cooking apple
> 6 tablespoons seedless raisins
> ½ cup chopped onion
> 2 tablespoons apple cider vinegar
> ¼ cup water
> 2 tablespoons Splenda Granular
> ½ teaspoon apple pie spice
> ¼ teaspoon table salt
> ¼ teaspoon black pepper
> 2 tablespoons Oscar Mayer or Hormel Real Bacon Bits

Spray a pressure cooker container with butter-flavored cooking spray. In prepared container, combine cabbage, apple, raisins, and onion. Stir in vinegar, water, Splenda, apple pie spice, salt, and black pepper. Place cover on cooker and bring to LOW pressure over medium heat. Lower heat to stabilize pressure and cook for 5 minutes. Remove from heat, wait for pressure to be released, and remove cover. Stir in bacon bits.

Each serving equals:

104 Calories • 0 gm Fat • 3 gm Protein • 23 gm Carbohydrate • 293 mg Sodium • 45 mg Calcium • 3 gm Fiber

DIABETIC EXCHANGES: 1 Fruit • 1 Vegetable

CARB CHOICES: 1½

Fruity Red Cabbage

This sweet side dish is wonderful with pork tenderloin and also looks great served at holiday time alongside a turkey or ham.

⏺ Serves 4 (1 cup)

> 3 cups chopped red cabbage
> 1 cup (1 medium) cored, peeled, and chopped cooking apple
> ¼ cup seedless raisins
> ½ cup chopped onion
> 1 tablespoon + 1 teaspoon I Can't Believe It's Not Butter!
>   Light Margarine
> 2 tablespoons apple juice
> ½ cup water
> ¼ cup Splenda Granular
> ½ teaspoon apple pie spice

Spray a pressure cooker container with butter-flavored cooking spray. In prepared container, combine cabbage, apple, raisins, onion, and margarine. Add apple juice, water, Splenda, and apple pie spice. Mix well to combine. Place cover on cooker and bring to LOW pressure over medium heat. Lower heat to stabilize pressure and cook for 5 minutes. Remove from heat, wait for pressure to be released, remove cover, and stir.

Each serving equals:

98 Calories • 2 gm Fat • 1 gm Protein • 19 gm Carbohydrate • 61 mg Sodium • 35 mg Calcium • 2 gm Fiber

---
DIABETIC EXCHANGES: 1 Fruit • 1 Vegetable

CARB CHOICES: 1

Cabbage and Mushroom Scallop

Scalloped vegetables are among my favorites to serve when guests come for Sunday lunch. They just seem more luxurious in their creamy coating.　　◐　　Serves 6 (½ cup)

> 6 cups shredded cabbage
> ¼ cup chopped onion
> ½ cup water
> 1 (10¾-ounce) can Healthy Request Cream of Mushroom
> 　　Soup
> 1 (2.5-ounce) jar sliced mushrooms, drained
> 2 tablespoons I Can't Believe It's Not Butter! Light
> 　　Margarine
> 1 (2-ounce) jar sliced pimiento, drained
> 1 teaspoon Worcestershire sauce

In a pressure cooker container, combine cabbage, onion, and water. Place cover on cooker and bring to LOW pressure over medium heat. Lower heat to stabilize pressure and cook for 5 minutes. Remove from heat, wait for pressure to be released, and remove cover. Drain and return cabbage mixture to pressure cooker container. Add mushroom soup, mushrooms, margarine, pimiento, and Worcestershire sauce. Mix well to combine. Cook over medium heat for 3 to 4 minutes, stirring often.

Each serving equals:

71 Calories • 3 gm Fat • 1 gm Protein • 10 gm Carbohydrate • 310 mg Sodium •
79 mg Calcium • 2 gm Fiber

DIABETIC EXCHANGES: 1 Vegetable • ½ Starch/Carbohydrate

CARB CHOICES: ½

Tossed Cabbage and Noodle Side Dish

In a fancy restaurant, there's someone on staff known as the "saucier," a person whose sole job is to prepare all the special sauces used in each dish. A pressure cooker is a little like having your own personal saucier, I think. ☻ Serves 4 (1 cup)

¾ cup water
4 cups coarsely chopped cabbage
½ cup chopped onion
1¾ cups uncooked medium egg noodles
1 (10¾-ounce) can Healthy Request Cream of Mushroom
    Soup
2 tablespoons I Can't Believe It's Not Butter! Light
    Margarine
¼ cup Land O Lakes Fat Free Half & Half
¼ cup Kraft Reduced Fat Parmesan Style Grated Topping
¼ teaspoon black pepper

In a pressure cooker container, combine water, cabbage, onion, and uncooked noodles. Evenly spread mushroom soup over noodle mixture to completely cover. Do not stir. Place cover on cooker and bring to LOW pressure over medium heat. Lower heat to stabilize pressure and cook for 8 minutes. Remove from heat, wait for pressure to be released, and remove cover. Add margarine, half & half, Parmesan cheese, and black pepper. Mix well to combine. Cook over medium heat for 2 to 3 minutes, stirring often.

Each serving equals:

185 Calories • 5 gm Fat • 5 gm Protein • 30 gm Carbohydrate • 499 mg Sodium • 131 mg Calcium • 3 gm Fiber

DIABETIC EXCHANGES: 2 Starch/Carbohydrate • 1 Vegetable • ½ Fat

CARB CHOICES: 2

Dill-Glazed Carrots

Even if the only garden you can grow is on your windowsill at home or at work, give it a try—and plant some fresh dill. It really adds a special touch to dishes, like this celebration of sweet carrots.

● Serves 4 (½ cup)

> *3 cups baby carrots*
> *½ cup water*
> *2 tablespoons I Can't Believe It's Not Butter! Light*
>   *Margarine*
> *2 tablespoons Splenda Granular*
> *1 tablespoon fresh dill weed or 1 teaspoon dried dill weed*

Spray a pressure cooker container with butter-flavored cooking spray. In prepared container, place carrots and water. Place cover on cooker and bring to LOW pressure over medium heat. Lower heat to stabilize pressure and cook for 2 minutes. Remove from heat, wait for pressure to be released, remove cover, and stir. Drain carrots. Melt margarine in cooker. Add Splenda, dill, and drained carrots. Mix well to combine. Cook over low heat for 2 to 3 minutes or until hot, stirring occasionally.

Each serving equals:

62 Calories • 2 gm Fat • 1 gm Protein • 10 gm Carbohydrate • 113 mg Sodium • 25 mg Calcium • 2 gm Fiber

DIABETIC EXCHANGES: 1½ Vegetable • ½ Fat

CARB CHOICES: ½

Calypso Carrots

Just as calypso music celebrates life with a joyful beat, so, too, does this lively carrot dish invite your taste buds to dance and sing! It's got great color—and great flavor, too! Serves 6 (⅓ cup)

3 cups diced carrots
½ cup chopped green bell pepper
¼ cup chopped red bell pepper
¾ cup chopped onion
1 tablespoon I Can't Believe It's Not Butter! Light Margarine
2 tablespoons white distilled vinegar
¼ cup water
¼ cup reduced-sodium ketchup
2 tablespoons Splenda Granular
½ teaspoon apple pie spice
¼ teaspoon black pepper

Spray a pressure cooker container with butter-flavored cooking spray. In prepared container, combine carrots, green pepper, red pepper, and onion. Add margarine, vinegar, water, ketchup, Splenda, apple pie spice, and black pepper. Mix well to combine. Place cover on cooker and bring to LOW pressure over medium heat. Lower heat to stabilize pressure and cook for 5 minutes. Remove from heat, wait for pressure to be released, remove cover, and stir.

Each serving equals:

61 Calories • 1 gm Fat • 1 gm Protein • 12 gm Carbohydrate • 70 mg Sodium • 30 mg Calcium • 2 gm Fiber

DIABETIC EXCHANGES: **2 Vegetable**

CARB CHOICES: **1**

Lyonnaise Carrots

This recipe evokes the spirit of Lyon, France, which is renowned for its rich potato dish cooked in butter. Here, I've taken that style of preparation and created a sunset-colored side dish that makes any dinner a party. ☾ Serves 4 (¾ cup)

> 4 cups fresh or frozen sliced carrots, thawed
> ½ cup chopped onion
> ½ cup water
> 2 tablespoons I Can't Believe It's Not Butter! Light
>   Margarine
> 2 teaspoons Splenda Granular
> 1 tablespoon chopped fresh parsley or 1 teaspoon dried
>   parsley flakes
> ¼ teaspoon table salt
> ¼ teaspoon black pepper

In a pressure cooker container, combine carrots, onion, and water. Place cover on cooker and bring to LOW pressure over medium heat. Lower heat to stabilize pressure and cook for 6 minutes. Remove from heat, wait for pressure to be released, and remove cover. Drain and return carrot mixture to pressure cooker container. Add margarine, Splenda, parsley, salt, and black pepper. Mix well to combine. Serve at once.

HINT: Thaw carrots by rinsing in a colander under hot water for 1
    minute.

Each serving equals:

87 Calories • 3 gm Fat • 1 gm Protein • 14 gm Carbohydrate • 302 mg Sodium • 49 mg Calcium • 3 gm Fiber

DIABETIC EXCHANGES: 2 Vegetable • ½ Fat

CARB CHOICES: 1

Orange-Glazed Carrots

Some vegetables, like these carrots, have a sensational sweet side, which makes them perfect for a fruity glaze! They offer a delightful sparkle and contrast when served with grilled meats.

☻ Serves 4 (½ cup)

> 3 cups fresh or frozen carrots, thawed
> ½ cup Diet Mountain Dew
> 3 tablespoons orange marmalade spreadable fruit
> 2 tablespoons Splenda Granular
> 2 tablespoons chopped walnuts

Spray a pressure cooker container with butter-flavored cooking spray. In prepared container, combine carrots and Diet Mountain Dew. Place cover on cooker and bring to LOW pressure over medium heat. Lower heat to stabilize pressure and cook for 5 minutes. Remove from heat, wait for pressure to be released, remove cover, and stir. Add spreadable fruit, Splenda, and walnuts. Cook over medium heat for 2 to 3 minutes, stirring often.

HINT: Thaw carrots by rinsing in a colander under hot water for 1 minute.

Each serving equals:

94 Calories • 2 gm Fat • 1 gm Protein • 18 gm Carbohydrate • 69 mg Sodium • 35 mg Calcium • 3 gm Fiber

DIABETIC EXCHANGES: 1½ Vegetable • ½ Fruit • ½ Fat

CARB CHOICES: 1

Carrot and Celery Scallop

It's a dieting cliché to snack on carrots and celery in their raw state, but I thought I'd demonstrate how succulent they can be when cooked "under pressure." ☻ Serves 6 (⅔ cup)

 3 cups diced carrots
 2 cups diced celery
 ½ cup chopped onion
 1 cup chopped fresh mushrooms
 1½ cups water
 3 tablespoons I Can't Believe It's Not Butter! Light
      Margarine
 2 teaspoons dried parsley flakes
 ¼ teaspoon black pepper

Spray a pressure cooker container with butter-flavored cooking spray. In prepared container, combine carrots, celery, onion, mushrooms, and water. Place cover on cooker and bring to LOW pressure over medium heat. Lower heat to stabilize pressure and cook for 6 minutes. Remove from heat, wait for pressure to be released, and remove cover. Drain and return vegetables to pressure cooker container. Add margarine, parsley flakes, and black pepper. Mix well to combine. Cook over low heat until hot, about 5 minutes, stirring occasionally.

Each serving equals:

67 Calories • 3 gm Fat • 1 gm Protein • 9 gm Carbohydrate • 145 mg Sodium • 43 mg Calcium • 2 gm Fiber

DIABETIC EXCHANGES: 2 Vegetable • ½ Fat

CARB CHOICES: ½

Sweet-and-Sour Carrots and Green Beans

How do you keep from getting bored with the same old vegetables? Simple—you jazz them up with a new way of cooking, like this one!   ☯   Serves 4 (1 cup)

> 2 cups fresh or frozen sliced carrots, thawed
> 1½ cups fresh or frozen cut green beans, thawed
> ½ cup chopped onion
> ½ cup water
> ¼ cup Splenda Granular
> 2 tablespoons apple cider vinegar
> ¼ teaspoon black pepper
> ¼ cup Oscar Mayer or Hormel Real Bacon Bits

In a pressure cooker container, combine carrots, green beans, onion, water, Splenda, vinegar, and black pepper. Place cover on cooker and bring to LOW pressure over medium heat. Lower heat to stabilize pressure and cook for 8 minutes. Remove from heat, wait for pressure to be released, remove cover, and stir. Drain and return mixture to pressure cooker container. Stir in bacon bits. Serve at once.

HINT: Thaw carrots and green beans by rinsing in a colander under hot water for 1 minute.

Each serving equals:

81 Calories • 1 gm Fat • 4 gm Protein • 14 gm Carbohydrate • 297 mg Sodium • 45 mg Calcium • 3 gm Fiber

DIABETIC EXCHANGES: 2 Vegetable • ½ Meat

CARB CHOICES: 1

Company Celery

Celery doesn't always get the respect it deserves, but this crunchy vegetable with lots of healthy fiber and a pretty pale green color is capable of so much more than many people believe! Try this dish and you'll be treating your family like company!

◐ Serves 4 (½ cup)

> 3 cups celery, cut into 1-inch pieces
> 1 (2-ounce) jar chopped pimiento, undrained
> 2 tablespoons water
> 2 tablespoons I Can't Believe It's Not Butter! Light
>   Margarine
> 1 tablespoon low-sodium soy sauce
> ¼ teaspoon black pepper

Spray a pressure cooker container with butter-flavored cooking spray. In prepared container, combine celery, undrained pimiento, water, margarine, soy sauce, and black pepper. Place cover on cooker and bring to LOW pressure over medium heat. Lower heat to stabilize pressure and cook for 4 minutes. Remove from heat, wait for pressure to be released, remove cover, and stir.

Each serving equals:

43 Calories • 3 gm Fat • 1 gm Protein • 3 gm Carbohydrate • 275 mg Sodium • 38 mg Calcium • 1 gm Fiber

DIABETIC EXCHANGES: 1 Vegetable • ½ Fat

CARB CHOICES: 0

Corn O'Brien

Want a pretty mélange of color on your supper plate? This dish of corn, pepper, and pimiento will light up the night!

○ Serves 4 (½ cup)

> 2 tablespoons I Can't Believe It's Not Butter! Light
>   Margarine
> ½ cup diced green bell pepper
> 2 cups fresh or frozen whole-kernel corn, thawed
> 1 (2-ounce) jar chopped pimiento, drained
> 3 tablespoons water
> ¼ teaspoon table salt
> ¼ teaspoon black pepper

Spray a pressure cooker container with butter-flavored cooking spray. In prepared container, melt margarine. Sauté green pepper for 2 minutes. Add corn, pimiento, water, salt, and black pepper. Mix well to combine. Place cover on cooker and bring to LOW pressure over medium heat. Lower heat to stabilize pressure and cook for 3 minutes. Remove from heat, wait for pressure to be released, remove cover, and stir.

HINT: Thaw corn by rinsing in a colander under hot water for 1 minute.

Each serving equals:

107 Calories • 3 gm Fat • 2 gm Protein • 18 gm Carbohydrate • 218 mg Sodium • 7 mg Calcium • 2 gm Fiber

DIABETIC EXCHANGES: 1 Starch • ½ Fat

CARB CHOICES: 1

Cheesy Creamed Corn

I know of similar recipes that use *tons* of cheese, but I'm happy to prove that it's not necessary to overload on cheese to get that cheesy-through-and-through flavor! ☛ Serves 6 (⅓ cup)

> 3 cups fresh or frozen whole-kernel corn, thawed
> ½ cup water
> ¼ cup Land O Lakes Fat Free Half & Half
> 2 tablespoons I Can't Believe It's Not Butter! Light
>   Margarine
> 1 tablespoon Splenda Granular
> ¼ teaspoon black pepper
> ¾ cup cubed Velveeta 2% Milk processed cheese
> 1 tablespoon chopped fresh parsley or 1 teaspoon dried
>   parsley flakes

In a pressure cooker container, combine corn and water. Place cover on cooker and bring to LOW pressure over medium heat. Lower heat to stabilize pressure and cook for 3 minutes. Remove from heat, wait for pressure to be released, and remove cover. Add half & half, margarine, Splenda, and black pepper. Mix well to combine. Stir in Velveeta cheese and parsley. Cook over medium heat for 3 to 4 minutes or until cheese melts, stirring often.

HINT: Thaw corn by rinsing in a colander under hot water for 1
    minute.

Each serving equals:

127 Calories • 3 gm Fat • 5 gm Protein • 20 gm Carbohydrate • 282 mg Sodium •
102 mg Calcium • 1 gm Fiber

DIABETIC EXCHANGES: 1 Starch • ½ Meat • ½ Fat

CARB CHOICES: 1

Comfort Corn and Potatoes

Corn and potatoes—two beloved starches—in the same dish? How decadent is that! But you can do it—and enjoy it—when you eat the Healthy Exchanges way. ☻ Serves 6 (½ cup)

2½ cups fresh or frozen whole-kernel corn, thawed
1 cup coarsely chopped raw potatoes
½ cup water
2 tablespoons I Can't Believe It's Not Butter! Light
    Margarine
1 tablespoon chopped fresh parsley or 1 teaspoon dried
    parsley flakes
¼ teaspoon black pepper

In a pressure cooker container, combine corn, potatoes, and water. Place cover on cooker and bring to LOW pressure over medium heat. Lower heat to stabilize pressure and cook for 6 minutes. Remove from heat, wait for pressure to be released, and remove cover. Drain and return vegetables to pressure cooker container. Add margarine, parsley, and black pepper. Mix well to combine. Serve at once.

HINT: Thaw corn by rinsing in a colander under hot water for 1 minute.

Each serving equals:

98 Calories • 2 gm Fat • 2 gm Protein • 18 gm Carbohydrate • 49 mg Sodium •
7 mg Calcium • 2 gm Fiber

DIABETIC EXCHANGES: 1 Starch • ½ Fat

CARB CHOICES: 1

Corn Spaghetti Side Dish

What a flavorful and fun use of this skinny pasta to create a combo with corn and cheese—yum, yum! It's delectably creamy and good to the last bite.   ☻   Serves 6 (⅓ cup)

1 cup broken uncooked spaghetti
1½ cups fresh or frozen whole-kernel corn, thawed
¼ cup chopped onion
⅛ teaspoon table salt
1½ cups water
2 tablespoons I Can't Believe It's Not Butter! Light
  Margarine
¼ cup Land O Lakes Fat Free Half & Half
¾ cup diced Velveeta 2% Milk processed cheese
1 teaspoon dried parsley flakes
¼ teaspoon black pepper

In a pressure cooker container, combine uncooked spaghetti, corn, onion, salt, and water. Place cover on cooker and bring to LOW pressure over medium heat. Lower heat to stabilize pressure and cook for 6 minutes. Remove from heat, wait for pressure to be released, and remove cover. Drain and return mixture to pressure cooker container. Stir in margarine and half & half. Add Velveeta cheese, parsley flakes, and black pepper. Mix well to combine. Cook over medium heat for 3 to 4 minutes or until cheese melts, stirring often.

HINT: Thaw corn by rinsing in a colander under hot water for 1 minute.

Each serving equals:

**123 Calories • 3 gm Fat • 5 gm Protein • 19 gm Carbohydrate • 330 mg Sodium •
103 mg Calcium • 1 gm Fiber**

DIABETIC EXCHANGES: 1 Starch • ½ Meat • ½ Fat

CARB CHOICES: 1

Comforting Green Beans with Almonds

I live with a green bean lover—and I bet you do, too! For him, and for everyone who loves this veggie in all its forms, here's a cozy, warm-your-heart version that offers just enough crunch to make you grin. ☻ Serves 4 (¾ cup)

4 cups fresh or frozen green beans, thawed
½ cup water
¼ teaspoon table salt
1 tablespoon + 1 teaspoon I Can't Believe It's Not Butter!
    Light Margarine
¼ cup blanched slivered almonds
1 tablespoon chopped fresh parsley or 1 teaspoon dried
    parsley flakes
¼ teaspoon black pepper

In a pressure cooker container, combine green beans, water, and salt. Place cover on cooker and bring to HIGH pressure over medium heat. Lower heat to stabilize pressure and cook for 3 minutes. Remove from heat, wait for pressure to be released, and remove cover. Drain beans. Melt margarine in cooker. Stir in almonds and sauté for 2 to 3 minutes. Add drained green beans, parsley, and black pepper. Mix well to combine. Continue cooking over low heat, uncovered, for 2 to 3 minutes, stirring often.

HINT: Thaw green beans by rinsing in a colander under hot water
    for 1 minute.

Each serving equals:

77 Calories • 3 gm Fat • 3 gm Protein • 11 gm Carbohydrate • 149 mg Sodium •
69 mg Calcium • 4 gm Fiber

DIABETIC EXCHANGES: 2 Vegetable • 1 Fat

CARB CHOICES: 1

Green Beans, Southern Style

I think southerners eat a bit more ham than the rest of the country, so it's not surprising to find bits of ham in this green bean side dish that would be welcome across those steamy states. Dishes like this ensure "the South will rise again!"   ☻   Serves 4 (1 cup)

> 4 cups fresh or frozen green beans, thawed
> 1 cup chopped onion
> ½ cup water
> ½ cup diced Dubuque 97% fat-free ham or any extra-lean ham
> ¼ teaspoon black pepper
> 1 teaspoon lemon pepper

Spray a pressure cooker container with butter-flavored cooking spray. In prepared container, combine green beans, onion, and water. Stir in ham and black pepper. Place cover on cooker and bring to LOW pressure over medium heat. Lower heat to stabilize pressure and cook for 10 minutes. Remove from heat, wait for pressure to be released, remove cover, and stir. Add lemon pepper. Mix well to combine.

HINT: Thaw green beans by rinsing in a colander under hot water for 1 minute.

Each serving equals:

64 Calories • 0 gm Fat • 5 gm Protein • 11 gm Carbohydrate • 277 mg Sodium • 63 mg Calcium • 4 gm Fiber

DIABETIC EXCHANGES: 2½ Vegetable • ½ Meat

CARB CHOICES: 1

Cliff's Savory Green Beans

My truck-drivin' man loves life on the spicy side, so adding chili sauce to green beans is his idea of heaven. I'm a wimp when it comes to heat, though, and this dish isn't too hot for me.

● Serves 6 (½ cup)

> 4 cups fresh or frozen cut green beans, thawed
> ½ cup chopped onion
> ½ cup water
> 1 tablespoon I Can't Believe It's Not Butter! Light Margarine
> ¼ cup Heinz Chili Sauce

In a pressure cooker container, combine green beans, onion, and water. Place cover on cooker and bring to HIGH pressure over medium heat. Lower heat to stabilize pressure and cook for 3 minutes. Remove from heat, wait for pressure to be released, and remove cover. Drain and return green bean mixture to pressure cooker container. Add margarine and chili sauce. Mix well to combine. Cook over medium heat for 2 to 3 minutes, stirring often.

HINT: Thaw green beans by rinsing in a colander under hot water for 1 minute.

Each serving equals:

53 Calories • 1 gm Fat • 1 gm Protein • 10 gm Carbohydrate • 27 mg Sodium • 40 mg Calcium • 2 gm Fiber

DIABETIC EXCHANGES: 2 Vegetable

CARB CHOICES: ½

Bacon-Flavored Green Beans

People ask me why I insist on using real bacon bits instead of the non-meat bits sold for topping salads. This is a perfect way to answer—by showing just how much a little *real* bacon does for a recipe.   ☻   Serves 8 (¾ cup)

½ cup chopped onion
2 tablespoons apple cider vinegar
⅓ cup water
2 teaspoons Splenda Granular
1 teaspoon dried parsley flakes
¼ teaspoon black pepper
6 cups frozen cut green beans, thawed
¼ cup Oscar Mayer or Hormel Real Bacon Bits

Spray a pressure cooker container with butter-flavored cooking spray. In prepared container, sauté onion for 5 minutes. Add vinegar, water, Splenda, parsley flakes, and black pepper. Mix well to combine. Stir in green beans. Place cover on cooker and bring to LOW pressure over medium heat. Lower heat to stabilize pressure and cook for 5 minutes. Remove from heat, wait for pressure to be released, remove cover, and stir. Stir in bacon bits.

HINT: Thaw green beans by rinsing in a colander under hot water for 1 minute.

Each serving equals:

57 Calories • 1 gm Fat • 3 gm Protein • 9 gm Carbohydrate • 128 mg Sodium • 42 mg Calcium • 2 gm Fiber

DIABETIC EXCHANGES: 1½ Vegetable

CARB CHOICES: ½

Special Green Beans

I like delivering more than I promise, so when I place this dish on the table, anyone who thinks it's just green beans will get a special surprise on first bite! The blend of horseradish and mustard gives these a piquant spark. ☻   Serves 6 (½ cup)

> 4 cups fresh or frozen cut green beans, thawed
> ½ cup chopped onion
> ½ cup water
> 2 tablespoons I Can't Believe It's Not Butter! Light
>   Margarine
> 1 tablespoon prepared yellow mustard
> 1 tablespoon prepared horseradish sauce
> ¼ teaspoon table salt
> ¼ teaspoon black pepper

In a pressure cooker container, combine green beans, onion, and water. Place cover on cooker and bring to HIGH pressure over medium heat. Lower heat to stabilize pressure and cook for 3 minutes. Remove from heat, wait for pressure to be released, and remove cover. Drain and return green bean mixture to pressure cooker container. Add margarine, mustard, horseradish sauce, salt, and black pepper. Mix well to combine. Cook over medium heat for 3 to 4 minutes or until beans are well coated, stirring often.

HINT: Thaw green beans by rinsing in a colander under hot water for 1 minute.

Each serving equals:

54 Calories • 2 gm Fat • 1 gm Protein • 8 gm Carbohydrate • 183 mg Sodium • 40 mg Calcium • 2 gm Fiber

DIABETIC EXCHANGES: 1½ Vegetable

CARB CHOICES: ½

Nutty Green Beans

I'm a nut about pecans, more than any other nut, and so even if I just get a spoonful or so in my serving, it still makes me happy— and satisfied. This dish has a zesty crunch I love.

◐ Serves 4 (½ cup)

> 1 tablespoon + 1 teaspoon I Can't Believe It's Not Butter!
>   Light Margarine
> ¼ cup chopped pecans
> 3 cups frozen cut green beans, thawed
> ⅓ cup water
> 1 teaspoon parsley flakes
> ¼ teaspoon black pepper

Spray a pressure cooker container with butter-flavored cooking spray. In prepared container, melt margarine. Stir in pecans and sauté for 2 to 3 minutes. Add green beans, water, parsley flakes, and black pepper. Mix well to combine. Place cover on cooker and bring to LOW pressure over medium heat. Lower heat to stabilize pressure and cook for 5 minutes. Remove from heat, wait for pressure to be released, remove cover, and stir.

HINTS: 1. Thaw green beans by rinsing in a colander under hot water for 1 minute.
2. To lower fat grams, use just 2 tablespoons pecans.

Each serving equals:

103 Calories • 7 gm Fat • 2 gm Protein • 8 gm Carbohydrate • 48 mg Sodium • 46 mg Calcium • 3 gm Fiber

DIABETIC EXCHANGES: 1½ Fat • 1½ Vegetable

CARB CHOICES: ½

Mom's Green Beans and Potatoes

My mother had a wonderful way with all kinds of dishes, and I learned so much by sitting in her kitchen and keeping my eyes and ears open. She could take a little of this and a little of that and produce something mouthwatering! Serves 6 (1 cup)

4 cups fresh or frozen cut green beans, thawed
3 cups peeled and diced raw potatoes
½ cup chopped onion
½ cup diced Dubuque 97% fat-free ham or any extra-lean ham
½ cup water
¼ teaspoon black pepper

Spray a pressure cooker container with butter-flavored cooking spray. In prepared container, combine green beans, potatoes, and onion. Stir in ham. Add water and black pepper. Mix well to combine. Place cover on cooker and bring to HIGH pressure over medium heat. Lower heat to stabilize pressure and cook for 5 minutes. Remove from heat, wait for pressure to be released, remove cover, and stir.

HINT: Thaw green beans by rinsing in a colander under hot water for 1 minute.

Each serving equals:

104 Calories • 0 gm Fat • 5 gm Protein • 21 gm Carbohydrate • 118 mg Sodium • 46 mg Calcium • 4 gm Fiber

DIABETIC EXCHANGES: 1½ Vegetable • 1 Starch

CARB CHOICES: 1½

Minted Peas

If you've got an herb garden, you may already have discovered which vegetables and meats go best with which herbs. If not, here's a good lesson—peas and mint are a superb "couple"!

◐ Serves 4 (½ cup)

> 2 cups fresh or frozen peas, thawed
> ¼ cup water
> 2 tablespoons I Can't Believe It's Not Butter! Light
>   Margarine
> 1½ teaspoons chopped fresh mint or ½ teaspoon dried mint
> ¼ teaspoon table salt
> ¼ teaspoon black pepper

In a pressure cooker container, combine peas and water. Place cover on cooker and bring to LOW pressure over medium heat. Lower heat to stabilize pressure and cook for 4 minutes. Remove from heat, wait for pressure to be released, and remove cover. Add margarine, mint, salt, and black pepper. Mix well to combine. Serve at once.

HINT: Thaw peas by rinsing in a colander under hot water for 1 minute.

Each serving equals:

79 Calories • 3 gm Fat • 3 gm Protein • 10 gm Carbohydrate • 294 mg Sodium • 17 mg Calcium • 3 gm Fiber

DIABETIC EXCHANGES: 1 Starch • ½ Fat

CARB CHOICES: ½

Baby Lima Beans and Tomatoes

The big lima beans aren't everyone's favorite veggie, but these baby ones are great. Blended with tomatoes and cooked under pressure, they are tender and terrific! ☻ Serves 6 (½ cup)

> 2 cups fresh or frozen baby lima beans, thawed
> ½ cup chopped onion
> 1 (15-ounce) can diced tomatoes, undrained
> ½ cup water
> 2 tablespoons I Can't Believe It's Not Butter! Light
>   Margarine
> 1 tablespoon Splenda Granular
> ¼ teaspoon black pepper

Spray a pressure cooker container with butter-flavored cooking spray. In prepared container, combine lima beans, onion, undrained tomatoes, and water. Add margarine, Splenda, and black pepper. Mix well to combine. Place cover on cooker and bring to LOW pressure over medium heat. Lower heat to stabilize pressure and cook for 9 minutes. Remove from heat, wait for pressure to be released, remove cover, and stir.

HINT: Thaw lima beans by rinsing in a colander under hot water for 1 minute.

Each serving equals:

81 Calories • 1 gm Fat • 3 gm Protein • 15 gm Carbohydrate • 222 mg Sodium • 28 mg Calcium • 4 gm Fiber

DIABETIC EXCHANGES: 1 Vegetable • ½ Starch

CARB CHOICES: 1

Butter Beans and Bacon

One of the best reasons to use a pressure cooker is to make magic with dried beans a lot more quickly. If you've never eaten butter beans, do give them a try. ☻ Serves 8 (¾ cup)

2 cups dried butter or lima beans
2 cups cold water
1 cup hot water
1 cup chopped onion
1 cup diced celery
1 (8-ounce) can tomatoes, chopped and undrained
1 tablespoon Splenda Granular
2 tablespoons I Can't Believe It's Not Butter! Light
   Margarine
6 tablespoons Oscar Mayer or Hormel Real Bacon Bits

In a large bowl, combine beans and cold water. Let set overnight or for at least 1 hour. Drain beans and rinse well. In a pressure cooker container, combine beans, hot water, onion, celery, undrained tomatoes, Splenda, and margarine. Place cover on cooker and bring to LOW pressure over medium heat. Lower heat to stabilize pressure and cook for 10 minutes. Remove from heat, wait for pressure to be released, remove cover, and stir. Just before serving, stir in bacon bits.

Each serving equals:

203 Calories • 3 gm Fat • 12 gm Protein • 32 gm Carbohydrate • 239 mg Sodium • 48 mg Calcium • 10 gm Fiber

DIABETIC EXCHANGES: 1½ Starch • 1 Meat • 1 Vegetable

CARB CHOICES: 1½

Party-Time Beans

Beans, beans, beans, beans—your can opener will get a workout, but it's worth every turn of the wrist! These look and taste amazing, so consider bringing them to your next potluck!

● Serves 8 (¾ cup)

> 1 cup chopped onion
> 1 (15-ounce) can kidney beans, rinsed and drained
> 1 (15-ounce) can great northern beans, rinsed and drained
> 1 (15-ounce) can butter or lima beans, rinsed and drained
> 1 (15-ounce) can black beans, rinsed and drained
> 1 (8-ounce) can Hunt's Tomato Sauce
> ¼ cup Splenda Granular
> 2 tablespoons white distilled vinegar
> 1½ teaspoons dried parsley flakes
> ¼ teaspoon black pepper

Spray a pressure cooker container with butter-flavored cooking spray. In prepared container, combine onion, kidney beans, great northern beans, butter or lima beans, and black beans. Add tomato sauce, Splenda, vinegar, parsley flakes, and black pepper. Mix well to combine. Place cover on cooker and bring to LOW pressure over medium heat. Lower heat to stabilize pressure and cook for 8 minutes. Remove from heat, wait for pressure to be released, remove cover, and stir.

Each serving equals:

136 Calories • 0 gm Fat • 8 gm Protein • 26 gm Carbohydrate • 151 mg Sodium • 64 mg Calcium • 7 gm Fiber

DIABETIC EXCHANGES: 1½ Starch • 1 Meat • ½ Vegetable

CARB CHOICES: 1

Baked Beans with Tomato Sauce

There are a million baked bean recipes out there (and quite a few are mine!), but I think this one, made with navy beans, is as tasty as it is inventive. The sauce is greater than all of its ingredients might suggest. ☻ Serves 8 (¾ cup)

2 cups dried navy beans
2 cups hot water
¼ cup minced onion
¼ cup Oscar Mayer or Hormel Real Bacon Bits
¼ cup Splenda Granular
3 cups water
¼ cup reduced-sodium ketchup
2 teaspoons prepared yellow mustard
1 (8-ounce) can Hunt's Tomato Sauce

In a large bowl, soak navy beans in hot water overnight or for at least 1 hour. Drain and rinse well. Spray a pressure cooker container with butter-flavored cooking spray. In prepared container, sauté onion for 2 to 3 minutes. Add beans, bacon bits, Splenda, water, ketchup, mustard, and tomato sauce. Mix well to combine. Place cover on cooker and bring to LOW pressure over medium heat. Lower heat to stabilize pressure and cook for 25 minutes. Remove from heat, wait for pressure to be released, remove cover, and stir.

Each serving equals:

209 Calories • 1 gm Fat • 13 gm Protein • 37 gm Carbohydrate • 291 mg Sodium • 83 mg Calcium • 13 gm Fiber

DIABETIC EXCHANGES: 2 Starch • 2 Meat • 1 Vegetable

CARB CHOICES: 1½

Boston Bean Pot

Beans have been a staple of New England cooking for centuries, and Boston beans have a taste all their own. The blend of molasses with the other ingredients is the magic key. ☻ Serves 8 (¾ cup)

> 2 *cups dried navy beans*
> 2 *cups cold water*
> 1 *cup diced onion*
> 4 *cups hot water*
> 1 *tablespoon vegetable oil*
> 2 *tablespoons Splenda Granular*
> ¼ *cup molasses*
> 1 *teaspoon prepared yellow mustard*
> 2 *tablespoons reduced-sodium ketchup*

In a large bowl, soak navy beans in cold water overnight or for at least 1 hour. Drain and rinse well. In a pressure cooker container, combine beans, onion, hot water, and vegetable oil. Place cover on cooker and bring to LOW pressure over medium heat. Lower heat to stabilize pressure and cook for 10 minutes. Remove from heat, wait for pressure to be released, and remove cover. Drain and return beans to pressure cooker container. Add Splenda, molasses, mustard, and ketchup. Mix well to combine.

Each serving equals:

230 Calories • 2 gm Fat • 11 gm Protein • 42 gm Carbohydrate • 14 mg Sodium • 103 mg Calcium • 13 gm Fiber

DIABETIC EXCHANGES: 2½ Starch • 1 Meat

CARB CHOICES: 2

Cliff's Veggie Side Dish

Sometimes I know when Cliff is coming home from the road, and sometimes he pops up unexpectedly. This is a dish I can make with little notice, using ingredients I always have on hand.

❂ Serves 4 (1 cup)

> 2 cups fresh or frozen cut green beans, thawed
> 2 cups fresh or frozen cut carrots, thawed
> 1 cup fresh or frozen whole-kernel corn, thawed
> ½ cup chopped onion
> ½ cup water
> 2 tablespoons I Can't Believe It's Not Butter! Light Margarine
> 1 teaspoon dried parsley flakes
> ¼ teaspoon lemon pepper

In a pressure cooker container, combine green beans, carrots, corn, onion, and water. Place cover on cooker and bring to LOW pressure over medium heat. Lower heat to stabilize pressure and cook for 6 minutes. Remove from heat, wait for pressure to be released, and remove cover. Drain and return vegetables to pressure cooker container. Add margarine, parsley flakes, and lemon pepper. Mix well to combine. Cook over medium heat for 2 to 3 minutes, stirring often.

HINT: Thaw green beans, carrots, and corn by rinsing in a colander under hot water for 1 minute.

Each serving equals:

115 Calories • 3 gm Fat • 2 gm Protein • 20 gm Carbohydrate • 141 mg Sodium • 56 mg Calcium • 5 gm Fiber

DIABETIC EXCHANGES: 2 Vegetable • ½ Starch • ½ Fat

CARB CHOICES: 1

Summer Garden Special

I'm so proud of my gardens, and so I love spending time every summer creating recipes that feature my glorious produce! This mélange of fresh flavors is delightful, whether you grow or buy your veggies. ☻ Serves 6 (1 cup)

> 3 cups fresh or frozen whole-kernel corn
> 2½ cups peeled and chopped fresh tomatoes
> 1 cup chopped unpeeled zucchini
> ½ cup finely chopped onion
> ¼ cup chopped green bell pepper
> ¼ cup chopped red bell pepper
> 2 tablespoons Splenda Granular
> 2 tablespoons chopped fresh basil or 1½ teaspoons dried
>   basil
> 1 tablespoon I Can't Believe It's Not Butter! Light Margarine

Spray a pressure cooker container with butter-flavored cooking spray. In prepared container, combine corn, tomatoes, zucchini, onion, green pepper, and red pepper. Stir in Splenda, basil, and margarine. Place cover on cooker and bring to LOW pressure over medium heat. Lower heat to stabilize pressure and cook for 5 minutes. Remove from heat, wait for pressure to be released, remove cover, and stir.

HINT: Thaw corn by rinsing in a colander under hot water for 1
    minute.

Each serving equals:

113 Calories • 1 gm Fat • 3 gm Protein • 23 gm Carbohydrate • 31 mg Sodium • 19 mg Calcium • 3 gm Fiber

DIABETIC EXCHANGES: 1 Starch • 1 Vegetable

CARB CHOICES: 1½

BBQ Onions

My friend Barbara is passionate about onions and loves to stir them into nearly every dish she makes. When she mentioned to me that she'd enjoyed a barbecue contest held in New York City, I was inspired to create this tangy side dish.

● Serves 6 (⅓ cup)

> 4½ cups coarsely chopped onion
> ½ cup water
> ¼ cup Healthy Choice Barbeque Sauce
> 2 tablespoons I Can't Believe It's Not Butter! Light
>   Margarine
> 1 tablespoon chopped fresh parsley or 1 teaspoon dried
>   parsley flakes

In a pressure cooker container, combine onion and water. Place cover on cooker and bring to LOW pressure over medium heat. Lower heat to stabilize pressure and cook for 20 minutes. Remove from heat, wait for pressure to be released, and remove cover. Drain and return onion to pressure cooker container. Stir in barbecue sauce, margarine, and parsley. Cook over medium heat for 2 to 3 minutes, stirring often.

Each serving equals:

74 Calories • 2 gm Fat • 1 gm Protein • 13 gm Carbohydrate • 134 mg Sodium • 30 mg Calcium • 1 gm Fiber

DIABETIC EXCHANGES: 2 Vegetable • ½ Fat

CARB CHOICES: 1

Homemade Stewed Tomatoes

Now, why would you stew tomatoes yourself when you can buy them quite inexpensively at any supermarket? One taste, and you'll see that there is just nothing like homemade. If you've got a big tomato harvest or picked up a basket at the farmer's market, you'll love this recipe. ☺ Serves 4 (¾ cup)

> 3 cups peeled and quartered fresh tomatoes
> ¾ cup finely chopped celery
> ¼ cup finely chopped onion
> 1 tablespoon chopped fresh parsley or 1 teaspoon dried
>   parsley flakes
> 1 tablespoon Splenda Granular
> ¼ teaspoon table salt
> ¼ teaspoon black pepper

Spray a pressure cooker container with butter-flavored cooking spray. In prepared container, combine tomatoes, celery, and onion. Add parsley, Splenda, salt, and black pepper. Mix well to combine. Place cover on cooker and bring to LOW pressure over medium heat. Lower heat to stabilize pressure and cook for 5 minutes. Remove from heat, wait for pressure to be released, remove cover, and stir.

Each serving equals:

32 Calories • 0 gm Fat • 1 gm Protein • 7 gm Carbohydrate • 170 mg Sodium • 26 mg Calcium • 2 gm Fiber

DIABETIC EXCHANGES: 1 Vegetable

CARB CHOICES: ½

Tomato Pasta Side Dish

Pasta makes a supremely satisfying accompaniment, especially when blended with vegetables—in this case both fresh and canned. Sometimes children who turn their noses up at eating their veggies will "miss" them in a plate of pasta.　　**○**　　Serves 6 (1 cup)

1 (15-ounce) can diced tomatoes, undrained
1 (8-ounce) can Hunt's Tomato Sauce
1 cup chopped celery
1 cup chopped onion
1¼ cups uncooked elbow macaroni
2 tablespoons Splenda Granular
1 cup water
1 teaspoon dried parsley flakes
¼ teaspoon black pepper

Spray a pressure cooker container with butter-flavored cooking spray. In prepared container, combine undrained tomatoes, tomato sauce, celery, and onion. Add uncooked macaroni, Splenda, water, parsley flakes, and black pepper. Mix well to combine. Place cover on cooker and bring to LOW pressure over medium heat. Lower heat to stabilize pressure and cook for 6 minutes. Remove from heat, wait for pressure to be released, remove cover, and stir.

Each serving equals:

108 Calories • 0 gm Fat • 4 gm Protein • 23 gm Carbohydrate • 305 mg Sodium • 29 mg Calcium • 2 gm Fiber

DIABETIC EXCHANGES: 1½ Vegetable • 1 Starch

CARB CHOICES: 1½

Macaroni and Tomatoes
à la Cleland

Cliff's dad, Cleland, is a pleasure to cook for, and over the years, he has sat at my table on many occasions. He likes macaroni in all its forms, from a cold salad to a hot entrée, and more. This recipe was inspired by my father-in-law's all-time favorite dish!

🍂 Serves 4 (¾ cup)

> 1 (15-ounce) can diced tomatoes, undrained
> ½ cup reduced-sodium tomato juice
> 1 tablespoon Splenda Granular
> 1 teaspoon dried parsley flakes
> ⅛ teaspoon black pepper
> 1 cup uncooked elbow macaroni
> ½ cup chopped onion
> 2 tablespoons I Can't Believe It's Not Butter! Light
>   Margarine

Spray a pressure cooker container with butter-flavored cooking spray. In prepared container, combine undrained tomatoes, tomato juice, Splenda, parsley flakes, and black pepper. Add uncooked macaroni, onion, and margarine. Mix well to combine. Place cover on cooker and bring to LOW pressure over medium heat. Lower heat to stabilize pressure and cook for 6 minutes. Remove from heat, wait for pressure to be released, remove cover, and stir.

Each serving equals:

159 Calories • 3 gm Fat • 4 gm Protein • 29 gm Carbohydrate • 280 mg Sodium • 32 mg Calcium • 3 gm Fiber

DIABETIC EXCHANGES: 1½ Starch • 1½ Vegetable. ½ Fat

CARB CHOICES: 2

Lemon Red Potatoes

It's remarkable that just a tablespoon of lemon juice can transform a dish of potatoes in wonderful ways! Look for the tiny red potatoes, as they are the best for this dish.   ☻   Serves 6 (⅔ cup)

1½ pounds small red potatoes, halved
½ cup water
3 tablespoons I Can't Believe It's Not Butter! Light
    Margarine
1 tablespoon lemon juice
2 teaspoons lemon pepper
¼ teaspoon table salt
¼ teaspoon black pepper

In a pressure cooker container, combine potatoes and water. Place cover on cooker and bring to LOW pressure over medium heat. Lower heat to stabilize pressure and cook for 12 minutes. Remove from heat, wait for pressure to be released, and remove cover. Drain and return potatoes to pressure cooker container. Add margarine, lemon juice, lemon pepper, salt, and black pepper. Mix well to combine. Serve at once.

Each serving equals:

84 Calories • 0 gm Fat • 2 gm Protein • 19 gm Carbohydrate • 249 mg Sodium •
12 mg Calcium • 2 gm Fiber

DIABETIC EXCHANGES: 1 Starch

CARB CHOICES: 1

Vegetable Medley

The more the merrier, they say, and it's all too true in this mélange of veggies, served in a festive sauce that celebrates tomatoes and dill. It's good all year round, too. ☾ Serves 4 (1 cup)

> 2 cups peeled and diced raw potatoes
> 1 cup fresh or frozen whole-kernel corn, thawed
> ¾ cup fresh or frozen sliced carrots, thawed
> ¼ cup chopped onion
> 1 (15-ounce) can diced tomatoes, undrained
> 2 tablespoons reduced-sodium ketchup
> 2 teaspoons Splenda Granular
> ¼ teaspoon dried dill weed
> ¼ teaspoon table salt
> ¼ teaspoon black pepper
> 2 tablespoons I Can't Believe It's Not Butter! Light
>   Margarine

Spray a pressure cooker container with butter-flavored cooking spray. In prepared container, combine potatoes, corn, carrots, onion, and undrained tomatoes. Stir in ketchup. Add Splenda, dill weed, salt, and black pepper. Mix well to combine. Place cover on cooker and bring to LOW pressure over medium heat. Lower heat to stabilize pressure and cook for 8 minutes. Remove from heat, wait for pressure to be released, remove cover, and stir. Stir in margarine. Serve at once.

HINT: Thaw corn and carrots by rinsing in a colander under hot water for 1 minute.

Each serving equals:

171 Calories • 3 gm Fat • 4 gm Protein • 32 gm Carbohydrate • 372 mg Sodium • 41 mg Calcium • 5 gm Fiber

DIABETIC EXCHANGES: 1½ Starch • 1½ Vegetable • ½ Fat

CARB CHOICES: 2

Potato Salad with Hot Dogs

Yes, you read the title of this recipe right—instead of hot dogs served with potato salad on the side, I'm serving potato salad with the dogs mixed right in! Don't they say that turnabout is fair play? Hurray!　　○　　Serves 6 (scant 1 cup)

4½ cups peeled and diced raw potatoes
8 ounces Oscar Mayer or Healthy Choice reduced-fat
  frankfurters, cut into bite-size pieces
3 tablespoons vegetable oil
3 tablespoons white distilled vinegar
1 cup water
2 tablespoons Splenda Granular
¼ teaspoon black pepper
¾ cup finely chopped onion
1 tablespoon chopped fresh parsley or 1 teaspoon dried
  parsley flakes

Spray a pressure cooker container with butter-flavored cooking spray. In prepared container, combine potatoes and frankfurters. Add vegetable oil, vinegar, water, Splenda, and black pepper. Mix well to combine. Stir in onion. Place cover on cooker and bring to HIGH pressure over medium heat. Lower heat to stabilize pressure and cook for 3 minutes. Remove from heat, wait for pressure to be released, remove cover, and stir. Stir in parsley.

Each serving equals:

200 Calories • 8 gm Fat • 7 gm Protein • 25 gm Carbohydrate • 391 mg Sodium • 19 mg Calcium • 2 gm Fiber

DIABETIC EXCHANGES: 1½ Starch • 1½ Fat • 1 Meat

CARB CHOICES: 1½

Potato Hot Dish Olé

Cooking with salsa saves the busy cook a lot of time, since someone else has already combined fresh veggies and spiced them as well. With the cheese and sour cream added, you'll think you're dining in your favorite Mexican taquería.　　●　Serves 8 (½ cup)

> 6 cups peeled and diced raw potatoes
> ¾ cup water
> 1 cup chunky salsa (mild, medium, or hot)
> 2 tablespoons + 2 teaspoons I Can't Believe It's Not Butter!
>　　Light Margarine
> 1 teaspoon dried parsley flakes
> ¼ teaspoon black pepper
> 1 cup cubed Velveeta 2% Milk processed cheese
> ½ cup Land O Lakes no-fat sour cream

In a pressure cooker container, combine potatoes and water. Place cover on cooker and bring to LOW pressure over medium heat. Lower heat to stabilize pressure and cook for 5 minutes. Remove from heat, wait for pressure to be released, and remove cover. Drain and return potatoes to pressure cooker container. Add salsa, margarine, parsley flakes, and black pepper. Mix well to combine. Stir in Velveeta cheese. Cook over medium heat for 4 to 5 minutes or until cheese melts, stirring often. Remove from heat. Add sour cream. Mix gently to combine. Serve at once.

Each serving equals:

151 Calories • 3 gm Fat • 5 gm Protein • 26 gm Carbohydrate • 527 mg Sodium • 116 mg Calcium • 2 gm Fiber

DIABETIC EXCHANGES: 1½ Starch/Carbohydrate • ½ Fat

CARB CHOICES: 2

Whipped Potatoes and Carrots

When I first began experimenting with fat-free half & half, I was astonished—and thrilled to find a product that was previously "off-limits" in my recipes because of the fat content of the original. Now I can create ultra-creamy dishes like this for all to enjoy!

○ Serves 4 (1 cup)

> 3 cups peeled and diced raw potatoes
> 1½ cups fresh or frozen chopped carrots, thawed
> ⅓ cup water
> ¼ teaspoon table salt
> 2 tablespoons I Can't Believe It's Not Butter! Light
>   Margarine
> ¼ cup Land O Lakes Fat Free Half & Half

In a pressure cooker container, combine potatoes, carrots, water, and salt. Place cover on cooker and bring to HIGH pressure over medium heat. Lower heat to stabilize pressure and cook for 5 minutes. Remove from heat, wait for pressure to be released, remove cover, and drain potatoes. Add margarine and half & half. Using a handheld electric mixer, whip mixture on HIGH speed for 1 to 2 minutes or until potatoes are fluffy. Serve at once.

HINT: Thaw carrots by rinsing in a colander under hot water for 1 minute.

Each serving equals:

139 Calories • 3 gm Fat • 3 gm Protein • 25 gm Carbohydrate • 268 mg Sodium • 54 mg Calcium • 3 gm Fiber

DIABETIC EXCHANGES: 1 Starch • 1 Vegetable • ½ Fat

CARB CHOICES: 1½

Creamed Potatoes and Peas

I first tried this recipe with fresh peas from the garden, just for fun, but it's fine with frozen peas as well. If you and your family love creamy mashed potatoes, this dish is for you.

Serves 6 (⅔ cup)

1½ cups fresh or frozen peas, thawed
2 cups peeled and cubed raw potatoes
1 cup water
1 (12-fluid-ounce) can Carnation Evaporated Fat Free Milk
3 tablespoons all-purpose flour
1 teaspoon dried parsley flakes
¼ teaspoon black pepper
1 tablespoon I Can't Believe It's Not Butter! Light Margarine

In a pressure cooker container, combine peas, potatoes, and water. Place cover on cooker and bring to LOW pressure over medium heat. Lower heat to stabilize pressure and cook for 6 minutes. Remove from heat, wait for pressure to be released, and remove cover. Drain and return vegetables to pressure cooker container. In a covered jar, combine evaporated milk, flour, parsley flakes, and black pepper. Shake well to blend. Pour milk mixture into potato mixture. Stir in margarine. Cook over medium heat for 4 minutes or until mixture thickens, stirring often.

HINT: Thaw peas by rinsing in a colander under hot water for 1 minute.

Each serving equals:

124 Calories • 0 gm Fat • 7 gm Protein • 24 gm Carbohydrate • 123 mg Sodium • 175 mg Calcium • 2 gm Fiber

DIABETIC EXCHANGES: 1½ Starch/Carbohydrate

CARB CHOICES: 1½

Majestic Mashed Potatoes

There are mashed potatoes, and then there are *mashed potatoes* "to die for!" With the addition of cream cheese, sour cream (fat-free but still luscious), and margarine, these potatoes are the stuff of dreams!   ☻   Serves 8 (½ cup)

> 6 cups peeled and chopped raw potatoes
> ¼ cup finely chopped onion
> ¾ cup water
> ½ cup (4 ounces) Philadelphia fat-free cream cheese, cubed
> ⅓ cup Land O Lakes no-fat sour cream
> 2 tablespoons + 2 teaspoons I Can't Believe It's Not Butter!
>   Light Margarine
> 1 teaspoon dried parsley flakes
> ¼ teaspoon black pepper

Spray a pressure cooker container with butter-flavored cooking spray. In prepared container, combine potatoes, onion, and water. Place cover on cooker and bring to LOW pressure over medium heat. Lower heat to stabilize pressure and cook for 10 minutes. Remove from heat, wait for pressure to be released, and remove cover. Drain and return mixture to pressure cooker container. Mash well with a potato masher. Add cream cheese, sour cream, and margarine. Mix well to combine. Stir in parsley flakes and black pepper. Serve at once.

Each serving equals:

122 Calories • 2 gm Fat • 4 gm Protein • 22 gm Carbohydrate • 150 mg Sodium • 29 mg Calcium • 2 gm Fiber

DIABETIC EXCHANGES: 1½ Starch/Carbohydrate • ½ Fat

CARB CHOICES: 1½

Sweet Potatoes
with Fruit & Nut Sauce

I've always felt that sweet potatoes loved being surrounded by sweet things, in part because they emerge from the ground sweeter than other potatoes. Crunchy, fruity, and impressively partnered with marshmallows, these potatoes are ready to party!

◐ Serves 4 (1¼ cups)

> 4 large sweet potatoes, peeled and quartered
> 1 cup water
> 2 tablespoons I Can't Believe It's Not Butter! Light Margarine
> 1 (8-ounce) can crushed pineapple, packed in fruit juice, undrained
> 1 tablespoon Splenda Granular
> ½ teaspoon ground cinnamon
> ¼ teaspoon ground nutmeg
> ½ cup miniature marshmallows
> ¼ cup chopped walnuts

Spray a pressure cooker container with butter-flavored cooking spray. In prepared container, combine sweet potatoes and water. Place cover on cooker and bring to LOW pressure over medium heat. Lower heat to stabilize pressure and cook for 6 minutes. Remove from heat, wait for pressure to be released, remove cover, and drain potatoes. Mash potatoes until fluffy. Add margarine, undrained pineapple, Splenda, cinnamon, and nutmeg. Mix well to combine. Stir in marshmallows and walnuts. Heat in cooker over low heat until hot, about 5 minutes, stirring occasionally.

Each serving equals:

209 Calories • 5 gm Fat • 3 gm Protein • 38 gm Carbohydrate • 77 mg Sodium • 59 mg Calcium • 5 gm Fiber

DIABETIC EXCHANGES: 2 Starch • 1 Fat • ½ Fruit

CARB CHOICES: 2

Sweet Potatoes Supreme

If you're eager to include fewer "white" foods in your daily menu for health reasons, here's another great recipe for moist and golden orange sweets—a delectable partner for plain or fancy entrées.

◐ Serves 4 (¾ cup)

> 3 cups peeled and chopped raw sweet potatoes
> ½ cup water
> 1 tablespoon + 1 teaspoon I Can't Believe It's Not Butter!
>   Light Margarine
> 2 tablespoons Splenda Granular
> 1 (8-ounce) can pineapple tidbits, packed in fruit juice,
>   drained and 2 tablespoons liquid reserved
> 2 tablespoons chopped pecans

In a pressure cooker container, combine sweet potatoes and water. Place cover on cooker and bring to LOW pressure over medium heat. Lower heat to stabilize pressure and cook for 8 minutes. Remove from heat, wait for pressure to be released, and remove cover. Drain and return sweet potatoes to pressure cooker container. Add margarine, Splenda, pineapple, and reserved pineapple liquid. Mix well to combine. Stir in pecans. Cook over medium heat for 2 to 3 minutes, stirring often.

HINT: If you can't find pineapple tidbits, use chunk pineapple and coarsely chop.

Each serving equals:

148 Calories • 4 gm Fat • 2 gm Protein • 26 gm Carbohydrate • 100 mg Sodium • 41 mg Calcium • 3 gm Fiber

DIABETIC EXCHANGES: 1 Starch • 1 Fat • ½ Fruit

CARB CHOICES: 2

Mushroom-Rice Side Dish

I've heard from some readers that they find rice "unexciting" or even bland. This makes sense to me, as rice straight from the pot is quite plain. Since at my house plain is never good enough, here's a scrumptious way to prepare rice that will make your taste buds sing!

◐ Serves 6 (½ cup)

> 2 tablespoons I Can't Believe It's Not Butter! Light
>   Margarine
> 2 cups chopped fresh mushrooms
> ½ cup chopped onion
> 1 (10¾-ounce) can Healthy Request Cream of Mushroom
>   Soup
> ¾ cup water
> 1 teaspoon Wyler's Reduced Sodium Beef Granules Instant
>   Bouillon
> ¼ teaspoon black pepper
> 1 cup uncooked Minute Rice

Spray a pressure cooker container with butter-flavored cooking spray. In prepared container, melt margarine. Stir in mushrooms and onion and sauté for 3 to 4 minutes. Add mushroom soup, water, dry bouillon, and black pepper. Mix well to combine. Stir in uncooked instant rice. Place cover on cooker and bring to LOW pressure over medium heat. Lower heat to stabilize pressure and cook for 4 minutes. Remove from heat, wait for pressure to be released, remove cover, and stir.

Each serving equals:

87 Calories • 3 gm Fat • 2 gm Protein • 13 gm Carbohydrate • 258 mg Sodium • 52 mg Calcium • 1 gm Fiber

DIABETIC EXCHANGES: 1 Starch • ½ Fat • ½ Vegetable

CARB CHOICES: 1

Spanish Rice on the Side

This speedy version of the popular classic is sure to appeal to the entire family. Vary the amount of chili seasoning if you like it a little hotter than we do!   ☻   Serves 4 (¾ cup)

½ cup finely chopped onion
½ cup finely chopped green bell pepper
1 (15-ounce) can diced tomatoes, undrained
1 cup water
1 cup uncooked Minute Rice
1 tablespoon Splenda Granular
1 teaspoon chili seasoning

Spray a pressure cooker container with butter-flavored cooking spray. In prepared container, brown onion and green pepper for 5 minutes. Stir in undrained tomatoes, water, and uncooked instant rice. Add Splenda and chili seasoning. Mix well to combine. Place cover on cooker and bring to LOW pressure over medium heat. Lower heat to stabilize pressure and cook for 5 minutes. Remove from heat, wait for pressure to be released, remove cover, and stir.

Each serving equals:

124 Calories • 0 gm Fat • 3 gm Protein • 28 gm Carbohydrate • 186 mg Sodium • 28 mg Calcium • 2 gm Fiber

DIABETIC EXCHANGES: 1½ Starch • 1 Vegetable

CARB CHOICES: 2

Spiced Acorn Squash

Winter squashes, especially acorn, do very well in the pressure cooker. But be very careful when cutting them in half, as they can easily roll and the knife may slip.   ☺   Serves 4 (1 cup)

> 2 small acorn squash, halved and seeds removed
> 1½ cups water
> ¼ cup Splenda Granular
> 1½ teaspoons apple pie spice
> 2 tablespoons I Can't Believe It's Not Butter! Light
>   Margarine
> ½ cup seedless raisins

In a pressure cooker container, place squash halves in bottom of pan. Pour water over top. Place cover on cooker and bring to LOW pressure over medium heat. Lower heat to stabilize pressure and cook for 10 minutes. Remove from heat, wait for pressure to be released, and remove cover. Drain. Scoop squash out of shells and place in a large bowl. Mash well with a potato masher. Add Splenda, apple pie spice, and margarine. Mix well to combine. Stir in raisins. Serve at once.

Each serving equals:

187 Calories • 3 gm Fat • 2 gm Protein • 38 gm Carbohydrate • 76 mg Sodium • 81 mg Calcium • 4 gm Fiber

DIABETIC EXCHANGES: 1 Starch • 1 Fruit • ½ Fat

CARB CHOICES: 2½

Magnificent

Main Dishes

When people ask, "What's for dinner?" they want to know about the entrée—the centerpiece of the delicious offerings from you, the chef of the evening. It's always a thrill to watch their faces when you announce the chosen dish. "Mmm-mm," they may say, or else just smile with anticipation. With the pressure cooker as your talented assistant, you're ready to stir up all kinds of excitement, whether you've invited the boss for dinner or planned a relaxing family feast before your favorite TV comedies begin.

Drumroll, please! You've got so many wonderful choices here, from the delightful informality of Chiligetti—*a funky combo of pasta and spicy beef—to more classic dinner-party fare, such as* Chicken Almondine with Rice. *You could dazzle the menfolk with* Steaks in Onion Gravy *or present American comfort food at its most delectable, with* Chicken-Macaroni Pot Pie. *And if everyone is just hungry, hungry, hungry, (warning: wordplay ahead), you could serve one of my new favorite dishes,* Hungarian Stew!

Creamy Fish Fillets

Pressure cooking produces a light and velvety fish entrée, in which all the herbs, spices, and cooking liquids combine for a luscious result. ☉ Serves 4

16 ounces whitefish, cut into 4 pieces
½ cup water
3 tablespoons I Can't Believe It's Not Butter! Light
  Margarine
3 tablespoons all-purpose flour
1 teaspoon dried dill weed
½ teaspoon dried minced garlic
¼ teaspoon lemon pepper
1 cup fat-free milk
¼ cup finely chopped green bell pepper
1 (2-ounce) jar chopped pimiento, drained

Spray a pressure cooker container with butter-flavored cooking spray. Arrange fish pieces in prepared container. Add water. Place cover on cooker and bring to LOW pressure over medium heat. Lower heat to stabilize pressure and cook for 6 minutes. Remove from heat, wait for pressure to be released, and remove cover. Drain and remove fish from cooker. Set aside. Melt butter in cooker container. Add flour, dill weed, garlic, lemon pepper, and milk. Mix well using a wire whisk. Stir in green pepper and pimiento. Cook over low heat until mixture thickens, stirring constantly using a wire whisk. Add fish pieces and heat.

Each serving equals:

173 Calories • 5 gm Fat • 23 gm Protein • 9 gm Carbohydrate • 198 mg Sodium • 85 mg Calcium • 0 gm Fiber

DIABETIC EXCHANGES: 3 Meat • 1 Fat • ½ Starch/Carbohydrate

CARB CHOICES: ½

Salmon Wild Rice Supper

Creamy rich and the palest of pinks, this nutritious and lovely dish is a superb choice for a busy weeknight when you don't want to fuss.

○ Serves 6 (⅔ cup)

> 1 (14.5-ounce) can pink salmon, drained, boned, and flaked
> 1 cup uncooked Minute Rice
> ½ teaspoon dried dill weed
> ¾ cup frozen peas, thawed
> 1½ cups water
> 1½ cups shredded fresh spinach leaves
> 6 tablespoons Land O Lakes no-fat sour cream

Spray a pressure cooker container with butter-flavored cooking spray. In prepared container, combine salmon, uncooked rice, dill weed, peas, and water. Place cover on cooker and bring to LOW pressure over medium heat. Lower heat to stabilize pressure and cook for 3 minutes. Remove from heat, wait for pressure to be released, remove cover, and stir. Add spinach and sour cream. Mix gently to combine. Serve at once.

HINT: Thaw peas by rinsing in a colander under hot water for 1 minute.

Each serving equals:

171 Calories • 3 gm Fat • 18 gm Protein • 18 gm Carbohydrate • 321 mg Sodium • 226 mg Calcium • 1 gm Fiber

DIABETIC EXCHANGES: 2 Meat • 1 Starch

CARB CHOICES: 1

Abram's Cheesy Tuna Noodle Scallop

Cooking with Grandma is one of Abram's favorite things to do, and this is his current favorite dish to share. He loves the little peas & carrots peeking out from the creamy tuna and noodles, and oh, how he loves cheese!   ☻   Serves 4 (1 cup)

1¼ cups uncooked noodles
1 (10¾-ounce) can Healthy Request Cream of Mushroom
     Soup
1 (6-ounce) can white tuna, packed in water, drained and
     flaked
¾ cup frozen peas & carrots, thawed
1 tablespoon I Can't Believe It's Not Butter! Light Margarine
1 teaspoon dried parsley flakes
¼ teaspoon black pepper
1½ cups water
½ cup cubed Velveeta 2% Milk processed cheese

Spray a pressure cooker container with butter-flavored cooking spray. In prepared container, combine uncooked noodles, mushroom soup, tuna, peas & carrots, margarine, parsley flakes, black pepper, and water. Place cover on cooker and bring to LOW pressure over medium heat. Lower heat to stabilize pressure and cook for 4 minutes. Remove from heat, wait for pressure to be released, remove cover, and stir. Add Velveeta cheese. Mix well to combine. Cook over medium heat for 3 to 4 minutes or until cheese melts, stirring often.

HINT: Thaw peas & carrots by rinsing in a colander under hot
     water for 1 minute.

Each serving equals:

266 Calories • 6 gm Fat • 18 gm Protein • 35 gm Carbohydrate • 729 mg Sodium • 164 mg Calcium • 2 gm Fiber

DIABETIC EXCHANGES: 2 Starch/Carbohydrate • 2 Meat

CARB CHOICES: 2

Grecian Shrimp and Rice

This Mediterranean-style supper takes you on a culinary sojourn to the Greek Islands—where the sun is bright, the water warm, and the food good enough for the gods of ancient Olympus. You can also prepare this with fresh cooked shrimp.

○ Serves 4 (¾ cup)

1 (6-ounce) package frozen shrimp, thawed
1 (15-ounce) can diced tomatoes, undrained
1 teaspoon oregano
1 tablespoon Splenda Granular
¼ cup feta cheese
1 cup uncooked Minute Rice
¾ cup water

Spray a pressure cooker container with olive oil–flavored cooking spray. In prepared container, combine shrimp, undrained tomatoes, oregano, Splenda, and feta cheese. Add uncooked instant rice and water. Mix well to combine. Place cover on cooker and bring to LOW pressure over medium heat. Lower heat to stabilize pressure and cook for 5 minutes. Remove from heat, wait for pressure to be released, remove cover, and stir.

Each serving equals:

175 Calories • 3 gm Fat • 12 gm Protein • 25 gm Carbohydrate • 304 mg Sodium • 90 mg Calcium • 2 gm Fiber

DIABETIC EXCHANGES: 2 Meat • 1 Starch • 1 Vegetable

CARB CHOICES: 1½

Shrimp Creole

In New Orleans, shrimp is a favorite entrée year round. The Creole style is a combination of Spanish cooking and island cuisine, richly flavored and savory.   ☉   Serves 4

> ¼ cup I Can't Believe It's Not Butter! Light Margarine
> 1 cup chopped onion
> ½ cup chopped celery
> 1 teaspoon minced garlic
> ½ cup chopped green bell pepper
> 2 (8-ounce) cans Hunt's Tomato Sauce
> 1 tablespoon fresh parsley or 1 teaspoon dried parsley flakes
> 1 bay leaf
> ½ cup water
> 2 (6-ounce) packages frozen shrimp, thawed
> 2 cups cooked rice

Spray a pressure cooker container with butter-flavored cooking spray. In prepared container, combine margarine, onion, celery, garlic, and green pepper. Sauté for 5 minutes. Stir in tomato sauce, parsley, bay leaf, water, and shrimp. Place cover on cooker and bring to LOW pressure over medium heat. Lower heat to stabilize pressure and cook for 8 minutes. Remove from heat, wait for pressure to be released, remove cover, and stir. Remove bay leaf. For each serving, place ½ cup rice on a plate and spoon 1 cup shrimp mixture over top.

HINT: Usually 1⅓ cups uncooked instant or 1 cup regular rice cooks to about 2 cups.

Each serving equals:

287 Calories • 7 gm Fat • 21 gm Protein • 35 gm Carbohydrate • 873 mg Sodium • 85 mg Calcium • 3 gm Fiber

DIABETIC EXCHANGES: 3 Meat • 2 Vegetable • 1½ Starch • ½ Fat

CARB CHOICES: 2

Spanish Rice Supper

This is one of my thriftier entrées, where a half pound of meat serves four people. How do I do it? By recognizing that if you blend the meat with lots of other tasty ingredients, you'll feel satisfied.

◐ Serves 4 (1 cup)

> *8 ounces extra-lean ground sirloin beef or turkey breast*
> *½ cup finely chopped onion*
> *½ cup finely chopped green bell pepper*
> *1 (15-ounce) can diced tomatoes, undrained*
> *½ cup reduced-sodium tomato juice*
> *½ cup water*
> *1 cup uncooked Minute Rice*
> *¼ cup Oscar Mayer or Hormel Real Bacon Bits*
> *1 teaspoon Italian seasoning*
> *1 teaspoon dried parsley flakes*
> *¼ teaspoon black pepper*

Spray a pressure cooker container with butter-flavored cooking spray. In prepared container, brown meat, onion, and green pepper. Stir in undrained tomatoes, tomato juice, water, uncooked instant rice, and bacon bits. Add Italian seasoning, parsley flakes, and black pepper. Mix well to combine. Place cover on cooker and bring to LOW pressure over medium heat. Lower heat to stabilize pressure and cook for 8 minutes. Remove from heat, wait for pressure to be released, remove cover, and stir.

Each serving equals:

203 Calories • 3 gm Fat • 14 gm Protein • 30 gm Carbohydrate • 473 mg Sodium • 31 mg Calcium • 2 gm Fiber

DIABETIC EXCHANGES: 2 Meat • 1½ Starch • 1½ Vegetable

CARB CHOICES: 2

Ranger Beans with Pasta

Once you stock your pantry with my favorite ingredients (especially varieties of canned beans and tomatoes), you can have supper on the table in no time at all! This dish is a great example—the only "fresh" items are a little beef and an onion.

◐ Serves 6 (1 cup)

> 8 ounces extra-lean ground sirloin beef or turkey breast
> ½ cup chopped onion
> 1 (8-ounce) can Hunt's Tomato Sauce
> ½ cup chunky salsa (mild, medium, or hot)
> 1¼ cups water
> 2 tablespoons Splenda Granular
> 1 (15-ounce) can Bush's butter beans, rinsed and drained
> 1 (15-ounce) can Bush's kidney beans, rinsed and drained
> 2½ cups uncooked noodles

Spray a pressure cooker container with butter-flavored cooking spray. In prepared container, brown meat and onion. Stir in tomato sauce, salsa, water, Splenda, butter beans, and kidney beans. Add uncooked noodles. Mix well to combine. Place cover on cooker and bring to LOW pressure over medium heat. Lower heat to stabilize pressure and cook for 5 minutes. Remove from heat, wait for pressure to be released, remove cover, and stir.

Each serving equals:

298 Calories • 2 gm Fat • 17 gm Protein • 53 gm Carbohydrate • 371 mg Sodium • 60 mg Calcium • 6 gm Fiber

DIABETIC EXCHANGES: 2 Meat • 2 Starch • 1 Vegetable

CARB CHOICES: 3

Italian Comfort Casserole

Wish you could bid *arrivederci* to all your troubles and just relax? Here's the dish to make that magic happen! Brimming with the flavors of *bella* Roma, this easy-to-fix main dish is sumptuous and soothing.   ☻   Serves 4 (1 cup)

> 8 ounces extra-lean ground sirloin beef or turkey breast
> ¼ cup chopped onion
> 1 (15-ounce) can diced tomatoes, undrained
> ½ cup water
> 1 (10¾-ounce) can Healthy Request Cream of Mushroom
>   Soup
> 1 (2.5-ounce) jar sliced mushrooms, drained
> 1 teaspoon Italian seasoning
> 1½ cups uncooked noodles
> ½ cup shredded Kraft reduced-fat mozzarella cheese
> ¼ cup Kraft Reduced Fat Parmesan Style Grated Topping

Spray a pressure cooker container with olive oil–flavored cooking spray. In prepared container, brown meat and onion. Stir in undrained tomatoes, water, mushroom soup, mushrooms, and Italian seasoning. Add uncooked noodles. Mix well to combine. Place cover on cooker and bring to LOW pressure over medium heat. Lower heat to stabilize pressure and cook for 3 minutes. Remove from heat, wait for pressure to be released, remove cover, and stir. Stir in mozzarella and Parmesan cheeses. Serve at once.

Each serving equals:

286 Calories • 6 gm Fat • 21 gm Protein • 37 gm Carbohydrate • 744 mg Sodium • 288 mg Calcium • 4 gm Fiber

DIABETIC EXCHANGES: 2 Meat • 2 Starch/Carbohydrate • 1 Vegetable

CARB CHOICES: 2½

Chiligetti

It sounds like the start of a joke: A bowl of chili was walking down the street when it crashed into a plate of spaghetti. A new specialty of the house was born: chiligetti!   ☻   Serves 6 (1 cup)

8 ounces extra-lean ground sirloin beef or turkey breast
½ cup chopped onion
½ cup chopped green bell pepper
1 (15-ounce) can diced tomatoes, undrained
1¼ cups water
1 (10¾-ounce) can Healthy Request Tomato Soup
1 tablespoon chili seasoning
1 (8-ounce) can red kidney beans, rinsed and drained
1⅓ cups broken uncooked spaghetti

Spray a pressure cooker container with butter-flavored cooking spray. In prepared container, brown meat and onion. Stir in green pepper, undrained tomatoes, water, tomato soup, chili seasoning, and kidney beans. Add uncooked spaghetti. Mix well to combine. Place cover on cooker and bring to LOW pressure over medium heat. Lower heat to stabilize pressure and cook for 5 minutes. Remove from heat, wait for pressure to be released, remove cover, and stir.

Each serving equals:

198 Calories • 2 gm Fat • 12 gm Protein • 33 gm Carbohydrate • 428 mg Sodium • 42 mg Calcium • 4 gm Fiber

DIABETIC EXCHANGES: 2 Starch • 1 Meat • 1 Vegetable

CARB CHOICES: 2

Cavatini Supper Pot

Here's a dish that demonstrates the magical powers of mozzarella cheese. All it requires is a little heat, and the cheese melts and stretches to perfection. Try not to get run over as your family races to the dinner table! ● Serves 4 (1 cup)

8 ounces extra-lean ground sirloin beef or turkey breast
1½ teaspoons Italian seasoning
1 (2.5-ounce) jar sliced mushrooms, drained
1 (15-ounce) can diced tomatoes, undrained
¾ cup water
1 teaspoon Splenda Granular
1½ cups uncooked rotini pasta
¾ cup shredded Kraft reduced-fat mozzarella cheese

Spray a pressure cooker container with butter-flavored cooking spray. In prepared container, brown meat. Stir in Italian seasoning and mushrooms. Add undrained tomatoes, water, Splenda, and uncooked rotini pasta. Mix well to combine. Place cover on cooker and bring to LOW pressure over medium heat. Lower heat to stabilize pressure and cook for 8 minutes. Remove from heat, wait for pressure to be released, remove cover, and stir. Stir in mozzarella cheese. Serve at once.

Each serving equals:

290 Calories • 6 gm Fat • 23 gm Protein • 36 gm Carbohydrate • 394 mg Sodium • 325 mg Calcium • 3 gm Fiber

DIABETIC EXCHANGES: 2 Meat • 2 Starch • 1 Vegetable

CARB CHOICES: 2

Beefy Noodle Pot

Do you remember how challenging it used to be to cook with bouillon cubes, those hard little nuggets that needed to be smashed with a spoon before you could use them? Well, no more, thanks to the good folks at Wyler's, whose granules *never* clump!

⊙ Serves 4 (¾ cup)

> 8 ounces extra-lean ground sirloin beef or turkey breast
> ½ cup finely chopped onion
> 1 (2.5-ounce) can sliced mushrooms, undrained
> 1 (10¾-ounce) can Healthy Request Cream of Mushroom
>   Soup
> 1½ teaspoons Wyler's Beef Granules Instant Bouillon
> ½ cup water
> 1½ cups uncooked noodles
> 1 teaspoon Worcestershire sauce
> ¼ teaspoon black pepper

Spray a pressure cooker container with butter-flavored cooking spray. In prepared container, brown meat and onion for 5 minutes. Stir in undrained mushrooms, mushroom soup, dry beef bouillon, and water. Add uncooked noodles, Worcestershire sauce, and black pepper. Mix well to combine. Place cover on cooker and bring to LOW pressure over medium heat. Lower heat to stabilize pressure and cook for 5 minutes. Remove from heat, wait for pressure to be released, remove cover, and stir.

Each serving equals:

265 Calories • 5 gm Fat • 17 gm Protein • 38 gm Carbohydrate • 443 mg Sodium • 78 mg Calcium • 2 gm Fiber

DIABETIC EXCHANGES: 2 Starch/Carbohydrate • 1½ Meat

CARB CHOICES: 2½

Beef and Green Bean Pot

So many people tell me that they struggle with figuring out the proper seasonings for a dish, and I answer that all cooks do. I just taste and test until I think I've got it right. Lemon pepper, mustard, tomato juice? That's it!   ☻   Serves 4 (1 cup)

> 8 ounces extra-lean ground sirloin beef or turkey breast
> ½ cup chopped onion
> 1 cup reduced-sodium tomato juice
> ½ cup water
> 1 teaspoon prepared yellow mustard
> 1 tablespoon Splenda Granular
> 1 teaspoon lemon pepper
> 2 cups frozen cut green beans, thawed
> 2 cups diced raw potatoes

Spray a pressure cooker container with butter-flavored cooking spray. In prepared container, brown meat and onion. Stir in tomato juice, water, mustard, Splenda, lemon pepper, green beans, and potatoes. Place cover on cooker and bring to LOW pressure over medium heat. Lower heat to stabilize pressure and cook for 6 minutes. Remove from heat, wait for pressure to be released, remove cover, and stir.

HINT: Thaw green beans by rinsing in a colander under hot water for 1 minute.

Each serving equals:

154 Calories • 2 gm Fat • 11 gm Protein • 23 gm Carbohydrate • 166 mg Sodium • 44 mg Calcium • 4 gm Fiber

DIABETIC EXCHANGES: 2 Vegetable • 1½ Meat • ½ Starch

CARB CHOICES: 1½

Welcome Home! Dinner Pot

Here's a dinner entrée so simple you can teach your teens how to make it, then enjoy the novelty of coming home one evening to a delicious aroma that says "Come on in!"

☻ Serves 6 (⅔ cup)

> 12 ounces extra-lean ground sirloin beef or turkey breast
> ½ cup chopped onion
> ½ cup chopped celery
> 1 (8-ounce) can Hunt's Tomato Sauce
> ¼ cup water
> 2 tablespoons Splenda Granular
> 2 tablespoons Worcestershire sauce
> 1 teaspoon chili seasoning
> 1 (15-ounce) can Bush's butter or lima beans, rinsed and
>   drained

Spray a pressure cooker container with butter-flavored cooking spray. In prepared container, brown meat, onion, and celery. Stir in tomato sauce, water, Splenda, Worcestershire sauce, and chili seasoning. Add beans. Mix well to combine. Place cover on cooker and bring to LOW pressure over medium heat. Lower heat to stabilize pressure and cook for 3 minutes. Remove from heat, wait for pressure to be released, remove cover, and stir.

Each serving equals:

114 Calories • 2 gm Fat • 11 gm Protein • 13 gm Carbohydrate • 318 mg Sodium • 33 mg Calcium • 2 gm Fiber

DIABETIC EXCHANGES: 2 Meat • 1 Vegetable • ½ Starch

CARB CHOICES: 1

Cliff's Sloppy Joes

This American classic never loses its charm, no matter where you go in the United States. I stirred up this version one night when Cliff was on his way home from the road, and I think it's got some extra pizzazz!   ●   Serves 6

16 ounces extra-lean ground sirloin beef or turkey breast
¾ cup chopped onion
¼ cup chopped green bell pepper
1 (15-ounce) can diced tomatoes, undrained
¼ cup water
1 tablespoon yellow prepared mustard
2 teaspoons Worcestershire sauce
¼ cup Quaker Old Fashioned Quick Oats
1 tablespoon Splenda Brown Sugar Blend
¼ teaspoon black pepper
6 small hamburger buns

Spray a pressure cooker container with butter-flavored cooking spray. In prepared container, brown meat, onion, and green pepper. Stir in undrained tomatoes, water, mustard, and Worcestershire sauce. Add oats, Splenda, and black pepper. Mix well to combine. Place cover on cooker and bring to LOW pressure over medium heat. Lower heat to stabilize pressure and cook for 5 minutes. Remove from heat, wait for pressure to be released, remove cover, and stir. For each sandwich, spoon a full ½ cup meat mixture between a hamburger bun.

Each serving equals:

196 Calories • 4 gm Fat • 17 gm Protein • 23 gm Carbohydrate • 343 mg Sodium • 23 mg Calcium • 2 gm Fiber

DIABETIC EXCHANGES: 2 Meat • 1 Starch • 1 Vegetable

CARB CHOICES: 1½

Comforting Tomato Beef Noodle Pot

Some foods just have the power to make us feel cozy and warm inside, and this beefy noodle dish does it every time! It's also extra easy, since everything goes straight into the pot.

○ Serves 6 (1 cup)

> 16 ounces extra-lean ground sirloin beef or turkey breast
> 1 (8-ounce) can Hunt's Tomato Sauce
> 1 (15-ounce) can diced tomatoes, undrained
> ¾ cup water
> 2 tablespoons Worcestershire sauce
> ½ cup chopped onion
> 1 (2.5-ounce) jar sliced mushrooms, drained
> 2½ cups uncooked noodles
> ¼ teaspoon black pepper

Spray a pressure cooker container with butter-flavored cooking spray. In prepared container, brown meat. Stir in tomato sauce, undrained tomatoes, water, and Worcestershire sauce. Add onion, mushrooms, uncooked noodles, and black pepper. Mix well to combine. Place cover on cooker and bring to LOW pressure over medium heat. Lower heat to stabilize pressure and cook for 5 minutes. Remove from heat, wait for pressure to be released, remove cover, and stir.

Each serving equals:

256 Calories • 4 gm Fat • 20 gm Protein • 35 gm Carbohydrate • 439 mg Sodium • 32 mg Calcium • 3 gm Fiber

DIABETIC EXCHANGES: 2 Meat • 2 Starch • 1½ Vegetable

CARB CHOICES: 3

Creole Stroganoff

Sometimes I think it would be fun to invite friends to a "stroganoff buffet," where I would serve lots of different versions of this creamy, dreamy dish. This one evokes memories of our visits to New Orleans before Hurricane Katrina.

● Serves 6 (1 cup)

> 16 ounces extra-lean ground sirloin beef or turkey breast
> ½ cup chopped onion
> ½ cup chopped green bell pepper
> 1 (14.5-ounce) can Hunt's Tomatoes Diced in Sauce
> 1 (10¾-ounce) can Healthy Request Cream of Mushroom Soup
> 1 teaspoon dried parsley flakes
> 1 tablespoon Splenda Granular
> ¼ teaspoon dried minced garlic
> 2½ cups uncooked noodles
> 1¼ cups water
> ¾ cup Land O Lakes no-fat sour cream

Spray a pressure cooker container with butter-flavored cooking spray. In prepared container, brown meat and onion for 5 minutes. Stir in green pepper, diced tomatoes, mushroom soup, parsley flakes, Splenda, and garlic. Add uncooked noodles and water. Mix well to combine. Place cover on cooker and bring to LOW pressure over medium heat. Lower heat to stabilize pressure and cook for 4 minutes. Remove from heat, wait for pressure to be released, remove cover, and stir. Stir in sour cream. Serve at once.

Each serving equals:

289 Calories • 5 gm Fat • 21 gm Protein • 40 gm Carbohydrate • 364 mg Sodium • 103 mg Calcium • 3 gm Fiber

DIABETIC EXCHANGES: 2 Meat • 2 Starch/Carbohydrate • 1 Vegetable

CARB CHOICES: 2½

Hearty Hamburger Casserole

This is one of those dishes that sends a clear message: Eat this, and you'll feel full! It's an old-fashioned meat-and-potatoes meal that will forever win the hearts of men! ☻ Serves 6 (1 full cup)

> 16 ounces extra-lean ground sirloin beef or turkey breast
> 1 (10¾-ounce) can Healthy Request Tomato Soup
> ¾ cup water
> 1½ teaspoons Wyler's Beef Granules Instant Bouillon
> 3 cups peeled and diced raw potatoes
> 1½ cups sliced fresh or frozen carrots, thawed
> 1 cup chopped celery
> ½ cup chopped onion
> ¼ teaspoon black pepper
> ¾ cup frozen peas, thawed

Spray a pressure cooker container with butter-flavored cooking spray. In prepared container, brown meat. Stir in tomato soup, water, and dry beef bouillon. Add potatoes, carrots, celery, onion, and black pepper. Mix well to combine. Place cover on cooker and bring to LOW pressure over medium heat. Lower heat to stabilize pressure and cook for 7 minutes. Remove from heat, wait for pressure to be released, remove cover, and stir. Stir in peas. Let set for 2 to 3 minutes. Gently stir again just before serving.

HINT: Thaw carrots and peas by rinsing in a colander under hot water for 1 minute.

Each serving equals:

212 Calories • 4 gm Fat • 18 gm Protein • 26 gm Carbohydrate • 278 mg Sodium • 39 mg Calcium • 4 gm Fiber

DIABETIC EXCHANGES: 2 Meat • 1 Starch • 1 Vegetable

CARB CHOICES: 2

Pizza Pot Casserole

When the kids ask why they can't order pizza to be delivered, smile and tell them, "This *is* pizza—but in a pot!" It's got all the flavors they love, and it's ready NOW. ☻ Serves 6 (1 cup)

> 16 ounces extra-lean ground sirloin beef or turkey breast
> 1 cup chopped onion
> 1 (15-ounce) can diced tomatoes, undrained
> ¼ cup water
> 1 (8-ounce) can Hunt's Tomato Sauce
> 1 (2.5-ounce) jar sliced mushrooms, drained
> 1 tablespoon Splenda Granular
> 1½ teaspoons pizza or Italian seasoning
> 2 cups uncooked rotini pasta
> ¾ cup shredded Kraft reduced-fat mozzarella cheese
> ¾ cup shredded Kraft reduced-fat Cheddar cheese

Spray a pressure cooker container with olive oil–flavored cooking spray. In prepared container, brown meat and onion. Stir in undrained tomatoes, water, tomato sauce, mushrooms, Splenda, and pizza seasoning. Add uncooked rotini pasta. Mix well to combine. Place cover on cooker and bring to LOW pressure over medium heat. Lower heat to stabilize pressure and cook for 5 minutes. Remove from heat, wait for pressure to be released, remove cover, and stir. Stir in mozzarella and Cheddar cheeses. Serve at once.

Each serving equals:

312 Calories • 8 gm Fat • 24 gm Protein • 36 gm Carbohydrate • 473 mg Sodium • 337 mg Calcium • 3 gm Fiber

DIABETIC EXCHANGES: 3 Meat • 1½ Starch • 1½ Vegetable

CARB CHOICES: 2½

Mom's Chop Suey

Originally, chop suey was a "kitchen sink" kind of dish, one in which you tossed all kinds of ingredients together in a pot. No one ingredient stood out, but together they produced a tasty meal. Here's one my mom would have been proud of!   ☻   Serves 6 (1 cup)

16 ounces extra-lean ground sirloin beef or turkey breast
1 cup uncooked Minute Rice
1 (15-ounce) can diced tomatoes, undrained
1½ cups water
2 cups finely shredded cabbage
1 cup chopped onion
½ cup chopped celery
1 tablespoon Splenda Granular
2 tablespoons reduced-sodium soy sauce
¼ teaspoon black pepper
¼ cup Oscar Mayer or Hormel Real Bacon Bits

Spray a pressure cooker container with butter-flavored cooking spray. In prepared container, brown meat. Stir in uncooked instant rice, undrained tomatoes, water, cabbage, onion, and celery. Add Splenda, soy sauce, and black pepper. Mix well to combine. Place cover on cooker and bring to LOW pressure over medium heat. Lower heat to stabilize pressure and cook for 6 minutes. Remove from heat, wait for pressure to be released, remove cover, and stir. Stir in bacon bits.

Each serving equals:

200 Calories • 4 gm Fat • 19 gm Protein • 22 gm Carbohydrate • 492 mg Sodium • 36 mg Calcium • 2 gm Fiber

DIABETIC EXCHANGES: 2 Meat • 1 Starch • 1 Vegetable

CARB CHOICES: 1½

Meat Loaf Meal

The pressure cooker is a kind of one-pot powerhouse, and this entrée is a good example of what it can do. Instead of juggling several pots on the stove, you prepare everything together!

◐ Serves 6

> 16 ounces extra-lean ground sirloin beef or turkey breast
> ½ cup finely chopped onion
> ½ cup finely chopped celery
> ½ cup grated carrots
> 10 Ritz Reduced Fat Crackers, made into crumbs
> ¼ cup chili sauce
> ½ teaspoon garlic powder
> ¼ teaspoon black pepper
> 1 tablespoon fresh parsley or 1 teaspoon dried parsley flakes
> 1 tablespoon vegetable oil
> 1 (10-ounce) package frozen peas, thawed
> 4 cups coarsely chopped raw potatoes
> 1 cup water

Spray a pressure cooker container with butter-flavored cooking spray. In a large bowl, combine meat, onion, celery, carrots, cracker crumbs, chili sauce, garlic powder, black pepper, and parsley. Mix well to combine. Using a ½ cup measuring cup as a guide, form mixture into 6 patties. Sprinkle vegetable oil in bottom of cooker container. Arrange patties in prepared container and brown for 3 minutes on each side. Remove patties from cooker. Evenly layer peas and potatoes in cooker container. Arrange browned patties over potatoes. Evenly pour water over top. Place cover on cooker and bring to LOW pressure over medium heat. Lower heat to stabilize pressure and cook for 8 minutes. Remove from heat, wait for pressure to be released, and remove cover. For each serving, place 1 patty on a plate and spoon about 1⅓ cups vegetables next to it.

HINT: Thaw peas by rinsing in a colander under hot water for 1 minute.

Each serving equals:

266 Calories • 6 gm Fat • 20 gm Protein • 33 gm Carbohydrate • 165 mg Sodium • 40 mg Calcium • 4 gm Fiber

DIABETIC EXCHANGES: 2 Meat • 2 Starch • ½ Fat

CARB CHOICES: 2

Hungarian Stew

Usually it's just one or two ingredients that place a dish in a particular culinary tradition, and this beefy stew is no exception. Why is it Hungarian? Paprika and caraway seeds! Enjoy.

☻ Serves 6

16 ounces extra-lean ground sirloin beef or turkey breast
¾ cup chopped onion
1 (15-ounce) can diced tomatoes, undrained
¾ cup water
2 tablespoons reduced-sodium ketchup
1 tablespoon paprika
1 teaspoon caraway seeds
½ teaspoon dried minced garlic
¼ teaspoon black pepper
2 teaspoons Splenda Granular
3 cups diced raw potatoes
¼ cup chopped green bell pepper
6 tablespoons Land O Lakes no-fat sour cream

Spray a pressure cooker container with butter-flavored cooking spray. In prepared container, brown meat and onion for 5 minutes. Add undrained tomatoes, water, ketchup, paprika, caraway seeds, garlic, black pepper, and Splenda. Mix well to combine. Stir in potatoes and green pepper. Place cover on cooker and bring to LOW pressure over medium heat. Lower heat to stabilize pressure and cook for 12 minutes. Remove from heat, wait for pressure to be released, remove cover, and stir. For each serving, spoon 1 cup stew mixture into a bowl and top with 1 tablespoon sour cream.

Each serving equals:

183 Calories • 3 gm Fat • 17 gm Protein • 22 gm Carbohydrate • 159 mg Sodium • 46 mg Calcium • 3 gm Fiber

DIABETIC EXCHANGES: 2 Meat • 1 Starch • 1 Vegetable

CARB CHOICES: 1½

Special Supper Pot

There are loads of good frozen entrées and prepackaged foods you could serve your family, but with my help, you can prepare a healthier, lower-sodium, homemade meal in about the same time, and often more cheaply. More than that, homemade says, "You're special!"   ☯   Serves 6 (1⅓ cups)

> 16 ounces extra-lean ground sirloin beef or turkey breast
> 1 cup chopped onion
> 3 tablespoons all-purpose flour
> 1 cup water
> 1 (15-ounce) can Bush's butter or lima beans, rinsed and
>   drained
> 1 (15-ounce) can diced tomatoes, undrained
> 1½ cups diced raw potatoes
> ¾ cup chopped celery
> ¾ cup chopped carrots
> 1 tablespoon Splenda Granular
> 2 teaspoons Worcestershire sauce
> ¼ teaspoon black pepper

Spray a pressure cooker container with butter-flavored cooking spray. In prepared container, brown meat and onion for 5 minutes. In a covered jar, combine flour and water. Shake well to blend. Add to browned meat. Mix well to combine. Stir in beans, undrained tomatoes, potatoes, celery, carrots, Splenda, Worcestershire sauce, and black pepper. Place cover on cooker and bring to LOW pressure over medium heat. Lower heat to stabilize pressure and cook for 6 minutes. Remove from heat, wait for pressure to be released, remove cover, and stir.

Each serving equals:

**188 Calories • 2 gm Fat • 15 gm Protein • 25 gm Carbohydrate • 167 mg Sodium •
51 mg Calcium • 5 gm Fiber**

DIABETIC EXCHANGES: 2½ Meat • 1½ Vegetable • 1 Starch

CARB CHOICES: 1

Spaghetti and Sauce Pot

Want an example of something you might not have thought to use your pressure cooker for? How about spaghetti and sauce? Instead of tending several pots on your stovetop, do it all at once—and do it beautifully! ☺ Serves 6 (1 cup)

> *16 ounces extra-lean ground sirloin beef or turkey breast*
> *1 cup chopped onion*
> *1 cup finely chopped fresh mushrooms*
> *1 (15-ounce) can diced tomatoes, undrained*
> *1 (8-ounce) can Hunt's Tomato Sauce*
> *1 cup reduced-sodium tomato juice*
> *1 tablespoon Splenda Granular*
> *1½ teaspoons Italian seasoning*
> *¼ teaspoon black pepper*
> *2 cups broken uncooked spaghetti*
> *6 tablespoons Kraft Reduced Fat Parmesan Style Grated*
> *   Topping*

Spray a pressure cooker container with olive oil–flavored cooking spray. In prepared container, sauté meat, onion, and mushrooms for 5 minutes. Add undrained tomatoes, tomato sauce, and tomato juice. Mix well to combine. Stir in Splenda, Italian seasoning, and black pepper. Add uncooked spaghetti. Mix well to combine. Place cover on cooker and bring to LOW pressure over medium heat. Lower heat to stabilize pressure and cook for 5 minutes. Remove from heat, wait for pressure to be released, remove cover, and stir. When serving, top each with 1 tablespoon Parmesan cheese.

Each serving equals:

267 Calories • 3 gm Fat • 18 gm Protein • 42 gm Carbohydrate • 515 mg Sodium • 31 mg Calcium • 4 gm Fiber

DIABETIC EXCHANGES: 2½ Meat • 1½ Starch • 1½ Vegetable

CARB CHOICES: 2

Sausage Supper Pot

Many people adore the flavor of sausage but are concerned about health issues when eating the real thing. If it's the flavor you love (and for me, it is), then let's cook up a tasty supper that tastes real but is much better for you!　❍　Serves 6 (1 cup)

> 16 ounces extra-lean ground sirloin beef or turkey breast
> 1 teaspoon poultry seasoning
> 1 teaspoon sage
> ¼ teaspoon garlic powder
> 2 cups unpeeled finely diced raw potatoes
> 1 cup chopped onion
> 1 (15-ounce) can whole-kernel corn, rinsed and drained
> ¾ cup water
> 1 (8-ounce) can Hunt's Tomato Sauce
> ¼ teaspoon black pepper

Spray a pressure cooker container with butter-flavored cooking spray. In prepared container, brown meat for 5 minutes. Stir in poultry seasoning, sage, and garlic powder. Add potatoes, onion, corn, water, tomato sauce, and black pepper. Mix well to combine. Place cover on cooker and bring to LOW pressure over medium heat. Lower heat to stabilize pressure and cook for 8 minutes. Remove from heat, wait for pressure to be released, remove cover, and stir.

Each serving equals:

191 Calories • 3 gm Fat • 14 gm Protein • 27 gm Carbohydrate • 235 mg Sodium • 23 mg Calcium • 3 gm Fiber

DIABETIC EXCHANGES: 2 Meat • 1 Starch • 1 Vegetable

CARB CHOICES: 2

Zucchini Supper Casserole

It's hearty, it's quick, and it's enough to make your mouth water in anticipation! Celebrate the bounties of the harvest with this marvelous meal-in-one-pot! ☻ Serves 8 (1 cup)

16 ounces extra-lean ground sirloin beef or turkey breast
½ cup chopped onion
1 cup diced carrots
3 cups diced unpeeled zucchini
1 (10¾-ounce) can Healthy Request Cream of Chicken
    Soup
1 (14-ounce) can Swanson Lower Sodium Fat Free Chicken
    Broth
1 teaspoon dried parsley flakes
½ cup Land O Lakes no-fat sour cream
3 cups herb-seasoned bread cubes

Spray a pressure cooker container with butter-flavored cooking spray. In prepared container, brown meat. Stir in onion, carrots, and zucchini. Add chicken soup, chicken broth, and parsley flakes. Mix well to combine. Place cover on cooker and bring to LOW pressure over medium heat. Lower heat to stabilize pressure and cook for 5 minutes. Remove from heat, wait for pressure to be released, remove cover, and stir. Just before serving, stir in sour cream and bread cubes.

Each serving equals:

175 Calories • 3 gm Fat • 13 gm Protein • 24 gm Carbohydrate • 401 mg Sodium • 41 mg Calcium • 2 gm Fiber

DIABETIC EXCHANGES: 1½ Meat • 1 Starch • 1 Vegetable

CARB CHOICES: 1½

Country-Style Beefsteaks

If you've traveled in the South, or eaten at country restaurants, you're probably familiar with a dish called Country Fried Steak. It's a deep-fried, crusty delight that is way too high in fat and calories for most of us to enjoy. But don't despair—here's a creative alternative that delivers the pleasure of the original! ☻ Serves 4

> 1 tablespoon + 1 teaspoon I Can't Believe It's Not Butter!
>   Light Margarine
> 1 egg, beaten, or equivalent in egg substitute
> ¾ cup dried bread crumbs
> 4 (4-ounce) lean minute beefsteaks
> 1 cup sliced onion
> ¼ cup water

Spray a pressure cooker container with butter-flavored cooking spray. Melt margarine in prepared container. Place egg in a saucer and bread crumbs in another. Dip each piece of steak first in egg, then in bread crumbs. Place coated steaks in prepared container. Brown steaks on low heat for 6 to 8 minutes on each side. Sprinkle onion slices over top. Pour water into pressure cooker container. Place cover on cooker and bring to LOW pressure over medium heat. Lower heat to stabilize pressure and cook for 12 minutes. Remove from heat, wait for pressure to be released, and remove cover. Serve at once.

Each serving equals:

268 Calories • 8 gm Fat • 31 gm Protein • 18 gm Carbohydrate • 264 mg Sodium • 58 mg Calcium • 1 gm Fiber

DIABETIC EXCHANGES: 3 Meat • 1 Starch • ½ Vegetable

CARB CHOICES: 1

Italian Swiss Steak

If you've ever been to the Vatican, you may know that the pope is protected by a private army called the Swiss Guards. But the Vatican is in Italy, right? Here's a dish that combines the Italian and Swiss styles of cooking! ◐ Serves 4

> 3 tablespoons all-purpose flour
> 1 teaspoon dried parsley flakes
> ¼ teaspoon black pepper
> 4 (4-ounce) tenderized lean minute steaks
> 1 cup sliced onion
> 1 cup diced celery
> ½ cup chopped green bell pepper
> ¼ cup reduced-sodium ketchup
> 1 tablespoon Italian seasoning
> 1 (15-ounce) can diced tomatoes, undrained
> ½ cup water

In a shallow saucer, combine flour, parsley flakes, and black pepper. Coat steaks in flour mixture. Spray a pressure cooker container with olive oil–flavored cooking spray. Arrange coated steaks in prepared container and brown for 2 to 3 minutes on each side. Sprinkle onion, celery, and green pepper evenly over meat. In a small bowl, combine ketchup, Italian seasoning, undrained tomatoes, and water. Spoon mixture over steaks. Place cover on cooker and bring to LOW pressure over medium heat. Lower heat to stabilize pressure and cook for 12 minutes. Remove from heat, wait for pressure to be released, and remove cover. When serving, spoon sauce evenly over top.

Each serving equals:

228 Calories • 4 gm Fat • 29 gm Protein • 19 gm Carbohydrate • 215 mg Sodium • 48 mg Calcium • 3 gm Fiber

DIABETIC EXCHANGES: 3 Meat • 2 Vegetable

CARB CHOICES: 1

Minute Steaks with Mushroom Gravy

My sons and grandsons have all been fans of those tender minute steaks you can find at your supermarket or big-box store. It doesn't take much to make those simple steaks spectacular—just some creamy gravy brimming with mushrooms! ☻ Serves 4

> 3 tablespoons all-purpose flour
> 1 teaspoon dried parsley flakes
> ¼ teaspoon black pepper
> 4 (4-ounce) tenderized lean minute steaks
> ½ cup fat-free milk
> 1 (10¾-ounce) can Healthy Request Cream of Mushroom Soup
> 1 (2.5-ounce) jar sliced mushrooms, undrained

In a shallow saucer, combine flour, parsley flakes, and black pepper. Coat steaks in flour mixture. Spray a pressure cooker container with butter-flavored cooking spray. Arrange steaks in prepared container and brown for 2 to 3 minutes on each side. Pour milk over steaks. In a medium bowl, combine mushroom soup, undrained mushrooms, and any remaining flour mixture. Spoon soup mixture over steaks. Place cover on cooker and bring to LOW pressure over medium-low heat. Lower heat to stabilize pressure and cook for 3 minutes. Remove from heat, wait for pressure to be released, and remove cover. For each serving, place 1 piece of steak on a plate and spoon mushroom gravy evenly over top.

Each serving equals:

213 Calories • 5 gm Fat • 29 gm Protein • 13 gm Carbohydrate • 431 mg Sodium • 102 mg Calcium • 1 gm Fiber

DIABETIC EXCHANGES: 3 Meat • 1 Starch/Carbohydrate

CARB CHOICES: 1

Steaks in Onion Gravy

It's good to have a repertoire of different sauces and gravies you can stir up quickly to serve over pastas and meats. This tangy blend turns the ordinary into something quite extraordinary—and in only minutes! ◐ Serves 4

3 tablespoons all-purpose flour
1 teaspoon dried parsley flakes
¼ teaspoon black pepper
4 (4-ounce) tenderized lean minute steaks
¾ cup water
1 cup finely chopped onion
1 (10¾-ounce) can Healthy Request Cream of Mushroom or
     Cream of Celery Soup

In a shallow saucer, combine flour, parsley flakes, and black pepper. Coat steaks in flour mixture. Spray a pressure cooker container with butter-flavored cooking spray. Arrange coated steaks in prepared container and brown for 2 to 3 minutes on each side. Pour water over browned steaks. In a medium bowl, combine onion, soup, and any remaining flour mixture. Spoon soup mixture over steaks. Place cover on cooker and bring to LOW pressure over medium heat. Lower heat to stabilize pressure and cook for 9 minutes. Remove from heat, wait for pressure to be released, and remove cover. When serving, spoon onion gravy evenly over steak pieces.

Each serving equals:

213 Calories • 5 gm Fat • 28 gm Protein • 14 gm Carbohydrate • 340 mg Sodium •
78 mg Calcium • 1 gm Fiber

DIABETIC EXCHANGES: 3 Meat • 1 Starch/Carbohydrate

CARB CHOICES: 1

Family's Choice Swiss Steak

Usually we test recipes on our Healthy Exchanges staff, but when we were tasting a group of entrée recipes, a number of family members stopped by. This was their number-one choice (among several), and so I've named it after that. ☯ Serves 4

6 tablespoons all-purpose flour
¼ teaspoon black pepper
16 ounces lean round steak, tenderized and cut into 4 pieces
1 tablespoon vegetable oil
1 cup chopped onion
¾ cup chopped celery
1 (15-ounce) can diced tomatoes, undrained
¼ cup water

In a saucer, combine flour and black pepper. Coat steak pieces in flour mixture. Spray a pressure cooker container with butter-flavored cooking spray. Sprinkle vegetable oil in bottom of cooker. Arrange meat in prepared container and brown steaks for 4 minutes on each side. In a medium bowl, combine onion, celery, undrained tomatoes, and water. Stir in any remaining flour mixture. Pour mixture over steaks. Place cover on cooker and bring to LOW pressure over medium heat. Lower heat to stabilize pressure and cook for 15 minutes. Remove from heat, wait for pressure to be released, and remove cover. When serving, spoon sauce evenly over steak pieces.

Each serving equals:

251 Calories • 7 gm Fat • 29 gm Protein • 18 gm Carbohydrate • 206 mg Sodium •
41 mg Calcium • 3 gm Fiber

DIABETIC EXCHANGES: 3 Meat • 2 Vegetable • 1 Starch

CARB CHOICES: 1

Mexican Beef and Beans

There is such an abundant choice on our market shelves, especially in the category of canned beans. Why use navy beans in this recipe and kidney beans in that one? It's a good question. I chose pinto beans here because they are so widely used in dishes created South of the Border! ◐ Serves 6 (1⅓ cups)

16 ounces lean round steak, tenderized and cut into bite-size pieces
1½ cups chopped onion
½ cup diced green bell pepper
2 (15-ounce) cans Bush's pinto beans, rinsed and drained
1 (15-ounce) can diced tomatoes, undrained
1 (8-ounce) can Hunt's Tomato Sauce
1 tablespoon Splenda Granular
1½ teaspoons chili seasoning

Spray a pressure cooker container with butter-flavored cooking spray. In prepared container, sauté steak pieces, onion, and green pepper for 5 minutes. Add pinto beans, undrained tomatoes, and tomato sauce. Mix well to combine. Stir in Splenda and chili seasoning. Place cover on cooker and bring to LOW pressure over medium heat. Lower heat to stabilize pressure and cook for 8 minutes. Remove from heat, wait for pressure to be released, remove cover, and stir.

Each serving equals:

256 Calories • 4 gm Fat • 30 gm Protein • 25 gm Carbohydrate • 383 mg Sodium • 59 mg Calcium • 6 gm Fiber

DIABETIC EXCHANGES: 3 Meat • 1 Starch • 1 Vegetable

CARB CHOICES: 1½

Connie's Pepper Beef

Peppers have always been considered an ideal complement to beef, and I think it's because they hold their own, don't get mushy (unless you really overcook them), and add strong flavor to the dish. This lively version of pepper steak was voted a success by everyone who tried it. ☻ Serves 6 (1 cup)

> 16 ounces lean round steak, tenderized and cut into bite-size pieces
> 2 ½ cups coarsely chopped green bell pepper
> 1 cup coarsely chopped onion
> 1 (8-ounce) can Hunt's Tomato Sauce
> 1 (15-ounce) can diced tomatoes, undrained
> 1 tablespoon Splenda Granular
> 1 tablespoon Worcestershire sauce
> ¼ teaspoon black pepper

Spray a pressure cooker container with butter-flavored cooking spray. In prepared container, sauté steak pieces, green pepper, and onion for 5 minutes. Add tomato sauce, undrained tomatoes, Splenda, Worcestershire sauce, and black pepper. Mix well to combine. Place cover on cooker and bring to LOW pressure over medium heat. Lower heat to stabilize pressure and cook for 15 minutes. Remove from heat, wait for pressure to be released, remove cover, and stir.

HINT: Great with pasta or rice.

Each serving equals:

184 Calories • 4 gm Fat • 25 gm Protein • 12 gm Carbohydrate • 364 mg Sodium • 35 mg Calcium • 3 gm Fiber

DIABETIC EXCHANGES: 2 Meat • 2 Vegetable

CARB CHOICES: 1

Mexican Beef Stew

Beef stew was (and continues to be) one of the most popular dishes prepared by people camping out or eating on the road. It's a dish that can cook for hours and not be ruined, it reheats well, and you can substitute ingredients without harming the end result. This savory version is popular with young and old.

● Serves 6 (1 cup)

> 16 ounces lean round or sirloin steak, tenderized and cut
>   into bite-size pieces
> ½ cup chopped onion
> ½ cup chopped green bell pepper
> 1 cup frozen whole-kernel corn, thawed
> 1 cup diced unpeeled raw potatoes
> 1 (8-ounce) can Hunt's Tomato Sauce
> 2 (14-ounce) cans Swanson Lower Sodium Fat Free Beef
>   Broth☆
> ½ cup chopped celery
> ½ cup chopped carrots
> 1 teaspoon chili seasoning
> 1 teaspoon dried parsley flakes
> ¼ teaspoon black pepper
> 3 tablespoons all-purpose flour

Spray a pressure cooker container with butter-flavored cooking spray. In prepared container, brown steak pieces for 5 minutes. Stir in onion, green pepper, corn, potatoes, and tomato sauce. Add 3¼ cups beef broth, celery, carrots, chili seasoning, parsley flakes, and black pepper. Mix well to combine. Place cover on cooker and bring to LOW pressure over medium heat. Lower heat to stabilize pressure and cook for 6 minutes. Remove from heat, wait for pressure to be released, remove cover, and stir. In a covered jar combine flour and remaining ¼ cup beef broth. Shake well to blend. Add to cooker and cook for 3 to 4 minutes, stirring often.

HINTS: 1. Thaw corn by rinsing in a colander under hot water for 1 minute.

2. Good served over biscuits.

Each serving equals:

220 Calories • 4 gm Fat • 27 gm Protein • 19 gm Carbohydrate • 425 mg Sodium • 25 mg Calcium • 2 gm Fiber

DIABETIC EXCHANGES: 2 Meat • 1 Starch • 1 Vegetable

CARB CHOICES: 1

Beef and Rice in Mushroom Gravy

I'm a big fan of the fat-free gravies you can purchase in jars at the supermarket. I know how hard it is to eliminate fat from home-made gravy, and this stuff tastes really good right from the jar. So when I add my personal touch, you get a dish that's lip-smacking good! ☻ Serves 4 (1 cup)

16 ounces lean round steak, tenderized and cut into bite-size
    pieces
½ cup chopped onion
1 (12-ounce) jar Heinz Fat Free Beef Gravy
1 cup water
1 (4-ounce) can sliced mushrooms, drained
1 cup uncooked Minute Rice
1 teaspoon dried parsley flakes
¼ teaspoon black pepper

Spray a pressure cooker container with butter-flavored cooking spray. In prepared container, sauté steak pieces and onion for 3 minutes. Add gravy, water, mushrooms, uncooked instant rice, parsley flakes, and black pepper. Mix well to combine. Place cover on cooker and bring to LOW pressure over medium heat. Lower heat to stabilize pressure and cook for 15 minutes. Remove from heat, wait for pressure to be released, remove cover, and stir.

HINT: Good served over potatoes or pasta.

Each serving equals:

309 Calories • 5 gm Fat • 39 gm Protein • 27 gm Carbohydrate • 689 mg Sodium • 20 mg Calcium • 1 gm Fiber

DIABETIC EXCHANGES: 3 Meat • 1½ Starch/Carbohydrate • ½ Vegetable

CARB CHOICES: 2

Beefy Stroganoff

Like any busy cook, I appreciate the convenience of veggies already cut up and ready to stir into my recipes. But in some dishes, fresh really matters, and that's why we're using fresh mushrooms here. Taste, texture, appearance—it's got it all!

○ Serves 6 (scant 1 cup)

16 ounces lean round steak, cut into bite-size pieces
2 cups chopped fresh mushrooms
½ cup chopped onion
1 (10¾-ounce) can Healthy Request Cream of Mushroom
  Soup
½ cup water
1½ teaspoons Wyler's Beef Granules Instant Bouillon
3 tablespoons all-purpose flour
¾ cup Land O Lakes no-fat sour cream
1 tablespoon chopped fresh parsley or 1 teaspoon dried
  parsley flakes

Spray a pressure cooker container with butter-flavored cooking spray. In prepared container, sauté steak pieces, mushrooms, and onion for 5 minutes. Stir in mushroom soup, water, and dry beef bouillon. Place cover on cooker and bring to LOW pressure over medium heat. Lower heat to stabilize pressure and cook for 12 minutes. Remove from heat, wait for pressure to be released, remove cover, and stir. Drain off ½ cup liquid. In a covered jar, combine drained liquid and flour. Shake well to blend. Add flour mixture, sour cream, and parsley to cooker. Mix well to combine. Cook over medium heat for 2 to 3 minutes or until mixture thickens, stirring often.

HINT: Great over noodles, potatoes, or toast.

Each serving equals:

180 Calories • 4 gm Fat • 26 gm Protein • 10 gm Carbohydrate • 109 mg Sodium • 50 mg Calcium • 0 gm Fiber

DIABETIC EXCHANGES: 2 Meat • ½ Starch/Carbohydrate • ½ Vegetable

CARB CHOICES: 1

Sweet-and-Sour Stew

Our tongues have special sensors that can distinguish sweet, sour, bitter, and salty, and most dishes emphasize one more than the others. But sometimes a combo of two is the best way to go, such as the sweet-and-sour sauce that ignites this glorious supper dish. ☻ Serves 8 (1 cup)

> 16 ounces lean round steak, cut into bite-size pieces
> 3 cups diced raw potatoes
> 1½ cups sliced carrots
> ½ cup chopped onion
> 1 cup chopped celery
> 1 (8-ounce) can Hunt's Tomato Sauce
> ¾ cup low-sodium tomato juice
> 1 cup water
> 2 tablespoons apple cider vinegar
> 1 teaspoon dried parsley flakes
> ¼ teaspoon black pepper

Spray a pressure cooker container with butter-flavored cooking spray. In prepared container, brown steak pieces for 5 minutes. Stir in potatoes, carrots, onion, and celery. Add tomato sauce, tomato juice, water, vinegar, parsley flakes, and black pepper. Mix well to combine. Place cover on cooker and bring to LOW pressure over medium heat. Lower heat to stabilize pressure and cook for 12 minutes. Remove from heat, wait for pressure to be released, remove cover, and stir.

Each serving equals:

142 Calories • 2 gm Fat • 15 gm Protein • 16 gm Carbohydrate • 252 mg Sodium • 31 mg Calcium • 2 gm Fiber

DIABETIC EXCHANGES: 1½ Meat • 1 Vegetable • ½ Starch

CARB CHOICES: 1

Belgian-Style Beef

It's a relatively small country, but it's had a pretty big influence on the flavors of food, from the famed sweet waffles to the twice-fried potatoes and, as demonstrated here, a tangy-sweet beer-based gravy for beef. The alcohol disappears during cooking, but the unique flavor remains. ☻ Serves 4 (¾ cup)

> 16 ounces lean round steak, tenderized and cut into large
>   bite-size pieces
> 1 cup coarsely chopped onion
> 1 (4-ounce) can sliced mushrooms, drained
> ½ cup non-alcoholic beer
> 2 tablespoons prepared yellow mustard
> ¼ teaspoon black pepper
> ½ cup seedless raisins

Spray a pressure cooker container with butter-flavored cooking spray. In prepared container, brown steak pieces and onion for 5 minutes. Add mushrooms, beer, mustard, black pepper, and raisins. Mix well to combine. Place cover on cooker and bring to LOW pressure over medium heat. Lower heat to stabilize pressure and cook for 12 minutes. Remove from heat, wait for pressure to be released, remove cover, and stir.

Each serving equals:

277 Calories • 5 gm Fat • 37 gm Protein • 21 gm Carbohydrate • 283 mg Sodium • 29 mg Calcium • 2 gm Fiber

DIABETIC EXCHANGES: 3 Meat • 1 Fruit • 1 Vegetable

CARB CHOICES: 1½

Pot Roast Perfecto

I could travel across America interviewing home cooks and come back with hundreds of recipes for the perfect pot roast. So when I call this dish "perfecto," it's with a bit of humility and a smile of pride. It's a goodie! ☺ Serves 6

    1 tablespoon vegetable oil
    2-pound lean boneless rolled beef rump roast
    1 cup sliced onions
    ½ cup coarsely chopped celery
    4 cups unpeeled raw potato chunks
    1 cup sliced carrots
    ½ teaspoon dried minced garlic
    1 teaspoon dried parsley flakes
    ¼ teaspoon black pepper
    1 (14-ounce) can Swanson Lower Sodium Fat Free Beef
        Broth

Heat vegetable oil in a pressure cooker container. Place beef roast in container and brown on all sides, about 8 to 10 minutes. Evenly layer onions, celery, potato chunks, and carrots over browned roast. Sprinkle garlic, parsley flakes, and black pepper over vegetables. Pour beef broth over top. Place cover on cooker and bring to LOW pressure over medium heat. Lower heat to stabilize pressure and cook for 30 minutes. Remove from heat, wait for pressure to be released, and remove cover. Remove roast and cut into 6 pieces. Stir vegetable mixture well. For each serving, place 1 piece of meat on a plate and spoon 1 cup vegetable mixture next to it.

Each serving equals:

254 Calories • 6 gm Fat • 28 gm Protein • 22 gm Carbohydrate • 193 mg Sodium • 35 mg Calcium • 3 gm Fiber

DIABETIC EXCHANGES: 3 Meat • 1 Starch • 1 Vegetable • ½ Fat

CARB CHOICES: 1½

Chicken-Macaroni Pot Pie

What dish is more comforting and cozy than a homemade chicken pot pie? From the time we are little, we learn to love chicken and veggies in a creamy sauce, right? Now you can enjoy those good memories in an extra-luscious version that substitutes macaroni for potatoes—yum! ☻ Serves 4 (1 cup)

> 8 ounces skinned and boned uncooked chicken breast, cut
>   into bite-size pieces
> 1 cup frozen cut carrots, thawed
> ½ cup frozen peas, thawed
> 1⅓ cups uncooked elbow macaroni
> 1 (10¾-ounce) can Healthy Request Cream of Chicken Soup
> 1 cup water
> 1 teaspoon dried parsley flakes
> 1½ teaspoons dried onion flakes
> ¼ teaspoon black pepper
> ¼ cup Land O Lakes no-fat sour cream
> ¼ cup Land O Lakes Fat Free Half & Half

Spray a pressure cooker container with butter-flavored cooking spray. In prepared container, sauté chicken pieces for 3 to 4 minutes. Stir in carrots, peas, uncooked macaroni, chicken soup, water, parsley flakes, onion flakes, and black pepper. Place cover on cooker and bring to LOW pressure over medium heat. Lower heat to stabilize pressure and cook for 5 minutes. Remove from heat, wait for pressure to be released, remove cover, and stir. Just before serving, stir in sour cream and half & half.

HINT: Thaw carrots and peas by rinsing in a colander under hot
    water for 1 minute.

Each serving equals:

**263 Calories • 3 gm Fat • 23 gm Protein • 36 gm Carbohydrate • 383 mg Sodium •
79 mg Calcium • 2 gm Fiber**

DIABETIC EXCHANGES: 2½ Starch/Carbohydrate • 1½ Meat • ½ Vegetable

CARB CHOICES: 2

Chicken Jambalaya

If you've never made it yourself, jambalaya is a rice dish with all the sizzle and heat of a Louisiana night on the bayou. This recipe uses chicken, but you can also do it with shrimp for a taste of New Orleans. It's all about the spices, *cher!* ☾ Serves 6 (1 cup)

8 ounces skinned and boned uncooked chicken breast, cut
into bite-size pieces
½ cup chopped onion
½ cup finely chopped celery
¼ cup chopped green bell pepper
1 (15-ounce) can diced tomatoes, undrained
1 (14-ounce) can Swanson Lower Sodium Fat Free Chicken
Broth
½ teaspoon dried minced garlic
1 teaspoon chili seasoning
¼ teaspoon cumin
¼ teaspoon Tabasco sauce
1 cup uncooked Minute Rice

Spray a pressure cooker container with butter-flavored cooking spray. In prepared container, sauté chicken pieces, onion, celery, and green pepper for 3 to 4 minutes. Stir in undrained tomatoes, chicken broth, garlic, chili seasoning, cumin, and Tabasco sauce. Add uncooked instant rice. Mix well to combine. Place cover on cooker and bring to LOW pressure over medium heat. Lower heat to stabilize pressure and cook for 5 minutes. Remove from heat, wait for pressure to be released, remove cover, and stir.

Each serving equals:

150 Calories • 2 gm Fat • 14 gm Protein • 19 gm Carbohydrate • 178 mg Sodium • 31 mg Calcium • 2 gm Fiber

DIABETIC EXCHANGES: 1 Meat • 1 Starch • 1 Vegetable

CARB CHOICES: 1

Chicken Almondine with Rice

Researchers tell us that almonds are a healthy nut and that it's good to include them in our menus on a regular basis. While snacking on them can lead to overeating, using them in a recipe is a smart way to enjoy just enough. ☻ Serves 4 (1 cup)

> 8 ounces skinned and boned uncooked chicken breast, cut
> into bite-size pieces
> ½ cup finely chopped onion
> ½ cup thinly sliced celery
> 1 (10¾-ounce) can Healthy Request Cream of Chicken
> Soup
> 1 cup water
> 1 teaspoon dried parsley flakes
> 1 cup uncooked Minute Rice
> ¼ cup Land O Lakes Fat Free Half & Half
> ¼ cup sliced almonds

Spray a pressure cooker container with butter-flavored cooking spray. In prepared container, sauté chicken pieces, onion, and celery for 3 to 4 minutes. Stir in chicken soup, water, and parsley flakes. Add uncooked instant rice. Mix well to combine. Place cover on cooker and bring to LOW pressure over medium heat. Lower heat to stabilize pressure and cook for 4 minutes. Remove from heat, wait for pressure to be released, remove cover, and stir. Stir in half & half and almonds.

Each serving equals:

266 Calories • 6 gm Fat • 21 gm Protein • 32 gm Carbohydrate • 338 mg Sodium • 72 mg Calcium • 2 gm Fiber

DIABETIC EXCHANGES: 2 Starch/Carbohydrate • 1½ Meat • ½ Fat

CARB CHOICES: 2

Linguine Chicken Primavera

Serve pasta with the flavor of spring, and every seat at your dining table will be filled! This is such an easy and pretty dish to serve, with the veggies providing lovely colors of red, green, and orange. *Delicioso!*   ☻   Serves 4 (¾ cup)

> *8 ounces skinned and boned uncooked chicken breast, cut*
> *into bite-size pieces*
> *1 cup chopped fresh broccoli*
> *½ cup chopped red bell pepper*
> *½ cup shredded carrots*
> *¾ cup water*
> *1 teaspoon Wyler's Chicken Granules Instant Bouillon*
> *½ teaspoon Italian seasoning*
> *1½ cups hot cooked linguine*
> *¼ cup Kraft Reduced Fat Parmesan Style Grated Topping*
> *¼ cup Land O Lakes Fat Free Half & Half*

Spray a pressure cooker container with olive oil–flavored cooking spray. In prepared container, combine chicken pieces, broccoli, red pepper, and carrots. Add water, dry chicken bouillon, and Italian seasoning. Mix well to combine. Place cover on cooker and bring to LOW pressure over medium heat. Lower heat to stabilize pressure and cook for 6 minutes. Remove from heat, wait for pressure to be released, remove cover, and stir. Add linguine, Parmesan cheese, and half & half. Mix well to combine. Serve at once.

HINT: Usually 1 cup broken uncooked linguine cooks to about 1½ cups.

Each serving equals:

218 Calories • 2 gm Fat • 21 gm Protein • 29 gm Carbohydrate • 202 mg Sodium • 51 mg Calcium • 2 gm Fiber

DIABETIC EXCHANGES: 2 Meat/Starch • 1 Vegetable

CARB CHOICES: 2

Zach's Oriental Chicken and Rice

My grandson Zach has loved being in the kitchen since he was old enough to sit on a stool and "hang out" with Grandma. He approved the rich and tangy sauce on the chicken in this dish, and he also liked the crunch of the water chestnuts.

☻ Serves 4 (1 cup)

> 8 ounces skinned and boned uncooked chicken breast, cut
>   into bite-size pieces
> 1 cup diagonal-cut celery
> ½ cup chopped onion
> 1 cup chopped fresh mushrooms
> 1 (8-ounce) can sliced water chestnuts, rinsed and drained
> 1 cup uncooked Minute Rice
> 1 (10¾-ounce) can Healthy Request Cream of Chicken
>   Soup
> 1 cup water
> ¼ cup reduced-sodium soy sauce

Spray a pressure cooker container with butter-flavored cooking spray. In prepared container, sauté chicken pieces for 3 minutes. Stir in celery, onion, mushrooms, water chestnuts, and uncooked instant rice. Add chicken soup, water, and soy sauce. Mix well to combine. Place cover on cooker and bring to LOW pressure over medium heat. Lower heat to stabilize pressure and cook for 5 minutes. Remove from heat, wait for pressure to be released, remove cover, and stir.

Each serving equals:

238 Calories • 2 gm Fat • 17 gm Protein • 38 gm Carbohydrate • 864 mg Sodium • 41 mg Calcium • 3 gm Fiber

DIABETIC EXCHANGES: 2 Starch/Carbohydrate • 1½ Meat • 1 Vegetable

CARB CHOICES: 2½

Chicken-Rice Stuffing Dish

For anyone who savors the special flavor of holiday stuffing, here's a dish that will bring back those splendid memories in each and every bite! The herbs and spices do the trick when blended with the chicken broth to create a wonderfully old-fashioned taste.

☻ Serves 6 (½ cup)

> *8 ounces skinned and boned uncooked chicken breast, cut into bite-size pieces*
> *1 cup chopped celery*
> *½ cup chopped onion*
> *1 (14-ounce) can Swanson Lower Sodium Fat Free Chicken Broth*
> *¼ teaspoon poultry seasoning*
> *1 teaspoon dried sage*
> *¼ teaspoon black pepper*
> *1 cup uncooked Minute Rice*

Spray a pressure cooker container with butter-flavored cooking spray. In prepared container, sauté chicken pieces, celery, and onion for 3 to 4 minutes. Stir in chicken broth, poultry seasoning, sage, and black pepper. Add uncooked instant rice. Mix well to combine. Place cover on cooker and bring to LOW pressure over medium heat. Lower heat to stabilize pressure and cook for 5 minutes. Remove from heat, wait for pressure to be released, remove cover, and stir.

Each serving equals:

130 Calories • 2 gm Fat • 13 gm Protein • 15 gm Carbohydrate • 62 mg Sodium • 22 mg Calcium • 0 gm Fiber

DIABETIC EXCHANGES: 1 Meat • 1 Starch

CARB CHOICES: 1

Chicken Supper Pot

For the creamiest, most luscious chicken dish, I'm starting with both a creamy soup and half & half. The sauce grabs hold of the noodles and never lets go! ☻ Serves 6 (⅔ cup)

> 16 ounces skinned and boned uncooked chicken breast, cut
>   into bite-size pieces
> 1 cup frozen peas & carrots, thawed
> 2 ¼ cups uncooked noodles
> 1 (10¾-ounce) can Healthy Request Cream of Chicken
>   Soup
> 1 cup water
> 1 teaspoon dried parsley flakes
> ¼ teaspoon black pepper
> ¼ cup Land O Lakes Fat Free Half & Half

Spray a pressure cooker container with butter-flavored cooking spray. In prepared container, sauté chicken pieces for 3 to 4 minutes. Stir in peas & carrots, uncooked noodles, chicken soup, water, parsley flakes, and black pepper. Place cover on cooker and bring to LOW pressure over medium heat. Lower heat to stabilize pressure and cook for 6 minutes. Remove from heat, wait for pressure to be released, remove cover, and stir in half & half. Serve at once.

HINT: Thaw peas & carrots by rinsing in a colander under hot
    water for 1 minute.

Each serving equals:

267 Calories • 3 gm Fat • 23 gm Protein • 37 gm Carbohydrate • 247 mg Sodium •
42 mg Calcium • 2 gm Fiber

DIABETIC EXCHANGES: 2½ Starch/Carbohydrate • 2 Meat

CARB CHOICES: 2½

Chicken Noodle Cacciatore

There's probably not an Italian restaurant anywhere in the United States that doesn't feature the renowned dish Chicken Cacciatore. The name actually translates as "hunter"-style, and it's traditionally made with tomato sauce and different veggies, all braised together. Adding noodles instead of spaghetti is a fun twist.

● Serves 6 (1 cup)

> 2 teaspoons olive oil
> 16 ounces skinned and boned uncooked chicken breast, cut
>   into bite-size pieces
> 1 (15-ounce) can diced tomatoes, undrained
> 1 (8-ounce) can Hunt's Tomato Sauce
> ¼ cup water
> 1 cup chopped onion
> ½ cup chopped green bell pepper
> 1 (2.5-ounce) jar sliced mushrooms, drained
> 1½ cups uncooked noodles
> ¼ cup sliced ripe olives
> 1½ teaspoons Italian seasoning
> 1 tablespoon Splenda Granular

Spray a pressure cooker container with olive oil–flavored cooking spray. Add olive oil and chicken pieces. Sauté chicken for 5 minutes. Add undrained tomatoes, tomato sauce, water, onion, green pepper, and mushrooms. Mix well to combine. Stir in uncooked noodles, olives, Italian seasoning, and Splenda. Place cover on cooker and bring to LOW pressure over medium heat. Lower heat to stabilize pressure and cook for 10 minutes. Remove from heat, wait for pressure to be released, remove cover, and stir.

Each serving equals:

240 Calories • 4 gm Fat • 21 gm Protein • 30 gm Carbohydrate • 425 mg Sodium • 41 mg Calcium • 3 gm Fiber

DIABETIC EXCHANGES: 2 Meat • 2 Vegetable • 1 Starch • ½ Fat

CARB CHOICES: 2

Easy Chicken and Veggies

I always try to offer you a bundle of chicken-based recipes in every one of my cookbooks. Poultry is still one of the best values, both nutritionally and for your pocketbook. I like this dish with peas and carrots, but it would also be great with green beans, or even a veggie blend.   ☻   Serves 6

16 ounces skinned and boned uncooked chicken breast, cut
    into bite-size pieces
½ cup chopped onion
1 (14-ounce) can Swanson Lower Sodium Fat Free Chicken
    Broth
1 cup frozen cut carrots, thawed
¾ cup frozen peas, thawed
1 teaspoon dried parsley flakes
½ teaspoon Wyler's Chicken Granules Instant Bouillon
5 tablespoons all-purpose flour

Spray a pressure cooker container with butter-flavored cooking spray. In prepared container, sauté chicken pieces and onion for 3 to 4 minutes. Stir in chicken broth, carrots, peas, parsley flakes, and dry chicken bouillon. Place cover on cooker and bring to LOW pressure over medium heat. Lower heat to stabilize pressure and cook for 6 minutes. Remove from heat, wait for pressure to be released, remove cover, and stir. Remove ½ cup hot liquid from cooker. In a covered jar, combine hot liquid and flour. Shake well to blend. Add mixture to cooker. Mix well to combine. Cook over medium heat for 3 to 4 minutes or until mixture thickens, stirring often.

HINT: Good served over biscuits or toast.

Each serving equals:

171 Calories • 3 gm Fat • 25 gm Protein • 11 gm Carbohydrate • 110 mg Sodium • 27 mg Calcium • 1 gm Fiber

DIABETIC EXCHANGES: 2 Meat • 1 Starch • ½ Vegetable

CARB CHOICES: 1

Hawaiian Chicken Supper Pot

Journey to the islands (without tangling with airport security or needing to unpack) by planning an informal luau tonight for family and friends! This is a colorful, tender, and flavorful dish, perfect for chasing the winter blues away. ☻ Serves 4 (1 cup)

> 16 ounces skinned and boned uncooked chicken breast, cut
>   into bite-size pieces
> 1½ cups chopped green bell pepper
> 1 cup sliced fresh mushrooms
> 1 (2-ounce) can chopped pimiento, undrained
> ¾ cup water
> 1 (15-ounce) can pineapple chunks, packed in fruit juice,
>   undrained
> 1 cup uncooked Minute Rice

Spray a pressure cooker container with butter-flavored cooking spray. In prepared container, sauté chicken pieces, green pepper, and mushrooms for 3 to 4 minutes. Stir in undrained pimiento, water, undrained pineapple, and uncooked instant rice. Place cover on cooker and bring to LOW pressure over medium heat. Lower heat to stabilize pressure and cook for 4 minutes. Remove from heat, wait for pressure to be released, remove cover, and stir.

Each serving equals:

267 Calories • 3 gm Fat • 28 gm Protein • 32 gm Carbohydrate • 61 mg Sodium • 39 mg Calcium • 2 gm Fiber

DIABETIC EXCHANGES: 3 Meat • 1 Fruit • 1 Starch • ½ Vegetable

CARB CHOICES: 2

Polynesian Chicken

Fruity sauces and chicken are a remarkably appetizing combination, and this recipe is both sweet and tangy when it's ready to serve. Make it fun by dressing your table with colorful linens or perhaps some festive flowers from your garden.

❂ Serves 4 (¾ cup)

> 16 ounces skinned and boned uncooked chicken breast, cut
>   into bite-size pieces
> ½ cup coarsely chopped onion
> 1 cup coarsely chopped green bell pepper
> 1 (8-ounce) can pineapple tidbits, packed in fruit juice,
>   undrained
> ½ cup unsweetened orange juice
> 2 teaspoons reduced-sodium soy sauce
> 1 teaspoon ground ginger
> ¼ cup slivered almonds
> ¼ cup flaked coconut

Spray a pressure cooker container with butter-flavored cooking spray. In prepared container, sauté chicken pieces, onion, and green pepper for 3 to 4 minutes. Add undrained pineapple, orange juice, soy sauce, and ginger. Mix well to combine. Place cover on cooker and bring to LOW pressure over medium heat. Lower heat to stabilize pressure and cook for 8 minutes. Remove from heat, wait for pressure to be released, remove cover, and stir. When serving, sprinkle 1 tablespoon almonds and 1 tablespoon coconut over top of each.

Each serving equals:

245 Calories • 9 gm Fat • 27 gm Protein • 14 gm Carbohydrate • 147 mg Sodium • 49 mg Calcium • 3 gm Fiber

DIABETIC EXCHANGES: 3 Meat • 1 Fruit • 1 Fat • ½ Vegetable

CARB CHOICES: 1

Apple-Cranberry Chicken Marsala

Marsala is actually an Italian dessert wine, originating in Sicily, but here I've created my own version of this sauce ingredient using fruit and juice. It's sweet and tart and pretty spectacular when you bring it to the table. ☻ Serves 4

> 2 tablespoons I Can't Believe It's Not Butter! Light
>   Margarine
> 16 ounces skinned and boned uncooked chicken breast, cut
>   into 4 pieces
> 1½ cups cored, peeled, and diced cooking apples
> ¼ cup dried cranberries
> ½ cup Ocean Spray reduced-calorie cranberry juice cocktail
> 2 tablespoons Splenda Granular
> 1 teaspoon dried parsley flakes

Spray a pressure cooker container with butter-flavored cooking spray. In prepared container, melt margarine. Place chicken pieces in prepared container and brown for 3 minutes on each side. Sprinkle apples and cranberries evenly over chicken. In a small bowl, combine cranberry juice cocktail, Splenda, and parsley flakes. Pour cranberry juice mixture evenly over top. Place cover on cooker and bring to LOW pressure over medium heat. Lower heat to stabilize pressure and cook for 8 minutes. Remove from heat, wait for pressure to be released, and remove cover. For each serving, place 1 piece of chicken on a plate and spoon a full ⅓ cup sauce mixture evenly over top.

Each serving equals:

209 Calories • 5 gm Fat • 25 gm Protein • 16 gm Carbohydrate • 123 mg Sodium • 18 mg Calcium • 1 gm Fiber

DIABETIC EXCHANGES: 3 Meat • 1 Fruit • ½ Fat

CARB CHOICES: 1

Chicken with Dijon Mustard Sauce

Does it actually make a difference which kind of mustard you use when you're cooking chicken? I think it does, which is why I call for Dijon style here. It's lighter than the prepared yellow mustard we grew up with, and yet it has a stronger flavor, which makes it great for cooking.   ❤   Serves 4

> ½ cup chopped onion
> 1 tablespoon olive oil
> 16 ounces skinned and boned uncooked chicken breast, cut
>   into 4 pieces
> ½ cup water
> 2 tablespoons Grey Poupon Country Style Dijon Mustard
> 1 teaspoon Wyler's Chicken Granules Instant Bouillon
> ¼ teaspoon black pepper
> 2 tablespoons all-purpose flour
> 2 tablespoons Land O Lakes Fat Free Half & Half

In a small skillet, sauté onion for 2 to 3 minutes in olive oil–flavored cooking spray. Pour olive oil into prepared pressure cooker container. Place chicken pieces in container and brown for 3 minutes on each side. Sprinkle sautéed onion evenly over chicken. In a small bowl, combine water, mustard, dry chicken bouillon, and black pepper. Pour mixture evenly over chicken. Place cover on cooker and bring to LOW pressure over medium heat. Lower heat to stabilize pressure and cook for 8 minutes. Remove from heat, wait for pressure to be released, and remove cover. In a covered jar, combine flour and half & half. Shake well to blend. Add flour mixture to cooker. Mix well to combine. Cook over medium heat for 3 to 4 minutes or until mixture thickens, stirring constantly. For each serving, place 1 piece of chicken on a plate and spoon about ¼ cup sauce mixture evenly over top.

Each serving equals:

**182 Calories • 6 gm Fat • 26 gm Protein • 6 gm Carbohydrate • 266 mg Sodium •
28 mg Calcium • 0 gm Fiber**

DIABETIC EXCHANGES: 3 Meat • 1 Fat

CARB CHOICES: ½

Chicken Fricassee

I read on the Internet that this dish was a thrifty favorite from the Depression years in America. It actually originated centuries ago in Europe and got its name from how the chicken is cut and prepared. Chicken Fricassee always produces a tender bird because of the long simmering process. ☾ Serves 4

16 ounces skinned and boned uncooked chicken breast, cut
into 4 pieces
1½ cups frozen sliced carrots, thawed
1 cup frozen peas, thawed
½ cup chopped onion
1 (10¾-ounce) can Healthy Request Cream of Chicken
Soup
¾ cup water
1 teaspoon Italian seasoning
2 teaspoons dried parsley flakes
3 tablespoons all-purpose flour

Spray pressure cooker container with butter-flavored cooking spray. Place chicken pieces evenly in prepared container and cook uncovered over medium heat for about 4 minutes on each side. Evenly sprinkle carrots, peas, and onion over chicken. In a small bowl, combine chicken soup, water, Italian seasoning, and parsley flakes. Pour mixture evenly over top. Place cover on cooker and bring to LOW pressure over medium heat. Lower heat to stabilize pressure and cook for 12 minutes. Remove from heat, wait for pressure to be released, and remove cover. Remove chicken pieces from cooker. Drain off ½ cup liquid. In a covered jar, combine liquid and flour. Shake well to blend. Add flour mixture to cooker. Cook over medium heat for 2 to 3 minutes or until mixture is thickened, stirring constantly. For each serving, place 1 piece of chicken on a plate and spoon 1 cup vegetable mixture next to it.

HINT: Thaw carrots and peas by rinsing in a colander under hot
water for 1 minute.

Each serving equals:

228 Calories • 4 gm Fat • 28 gm Protein • 20 gm Carbohydrate • 399 mg Sodium • 46 mg Calcium • 3 gm Fiber

DIABETIC EXCHANGES: 3 Meat • 1 Starch/Carbohydrate • 1 Vegetable

CARB CHOICES: 1

Chicken and Rice à la Orange

This is such a pretty dish, you might want to save it just for dinner parties—but don't! Your family will love it and it's so easy to do, you'll make it all the time. The orange flavor really gets into the chicken and makes it tender-sweet. ● Serves 4

> ¼ cup sliced almonds
> 16 ounces skinned and boned uncooked chicken breast, cut into 4 pieces
> 1 cup uncooked Minute Rice
> 1 cup unsweetened orange juice
> 1 tablespoon + 1 teaspoon I Can't Believe It's Not Butter! Light Margarine
> 3 tablespoons orange marmalade spreadable fruit

Spray a pressure cooker container with butter-flavored cooking spray. In prepared container, sauté almonds for 1 to 2 minutes. Add chicken pieces and brown for 3 minutes on each side. Stir in uncooked instant rice, orange juice, margarine, and spreadable fruit. Place cover on cooker and bring to LOW pressure over medium heat. Lower heat to stabilize pressure and cook for 8 minutes. Remove from heat, wait for pressure to be released, and remove cover. For each serving, place 1 piece of chicken on a plate and spoon about ½ cup rice mixture next to it.

Each serving equals:

320 Calories • 8 gm Fat • 28 gm Protein • 34 gm Carbohydrate • 102 mg Sodium • 40 mg Calcium • 1 gm Fiber

DIABETIC EXCHANGES: 3 Meat • 1 Starch • 1 Fruit • 1 Fat

CARB CHOICES: 2

Chicken Veronique

Even if you think French cuisine is way too fancy for your taste buds, I hope you will give this recipe a chance. *Veronique* means "with grapes," and if you can't find white grapes, green would be okay, too. The grape juice enhances the flavor.

● Serves 4

> 1 tablespoon + 1 teaspoon I Can't Believe It's Not Butter!
>   Light Margarine
> 16 ounces skinned and boned uncooked chicken breast, cut
>   into 4 pieces
> ⅓ cup white grape juice
> 1 cup water☆
> 1 teaspoon Wyler's Chicken Granules Instant Bouillon
> 3 tablespoons cornstarch
> 1 cup seedless white grapes

Spray a pressure cooker container with butter-flavored cooking spray. In prepared container, melt margarine. Brown chicken pieces in prepared container for 3 minutes on each side. In a medium bowl, combine grape juice, ¾ cup water, and dry chicken bouillon. Mix well using a wire whisk. Pour mixture evenly over chicken pieces. Place cover on cooker and bring to LOW pressure over medium heat. Lower heat to stabilize pressure and cook for 6 minutes. Remove from heat, wait for pressure to be released, and remove cover. In a covered jar, combine remaining ¼ cup water and cornstarch. Shake well to blend. Add cornstarch mixture to cooker. Cook over medium heat for 2 to 3 minutes or until mixture thickens, stirring constantly using a wire whisk. Stir in grapes. Let set for 2 minutes. For each serving, place 1 piece of chicken on a plate and spoon about ½ cup sauce mixture evenly over top.

Each serving equals:

200 Calories • 4 gm Fat • 25 gm Protein • 16 gm Carbohydrate • 126 mg Sodium • 19 mg Calcium • 0 gm Fiber

DIABETIC EXCHANGES: 3 Meat • ½ Starch • ½ Fruit • ½ Fat

CARB CHOICES: 1

Near-Perfect Fried Chicken

What would make this perfect, you ask? Well, the perfect stuff is golden-crusted, fried in oil, and not at all healthy—but delicious. This is almost that good, and it's good for you, so that's great!

☻ Serves 4

> 6 tablespoons all-purpose flour
> ¼ teaspoon black pepper
> 1 tablespoon paprika
> 16 ounces skinned and boned uncooked chicken breast, cut
>   into 4 pieces
> 2 teaspoons I Can't Believe It's Not Butter! Light Margarine
> 1 tablespoon vegetable oil

In a shallow saucer, combine flour, black pepper, and paprika. Coat chicken pieces in flour mixture. In a pressure cooker container, melt margarine. Arrange chicken pieces in container and brown for 2 minutes on each side. Sprinkle vegetable oil evenly over chicken pieces. Place cover on cooker and bring to LOW pressure over medium heat. Lower heat to stabilize pressure and cook for 10 minutes. Remove from heat, wait for pressure to be released, and remove cover.

Each serving equals:

169 Calories • 5 gm Fat • 21 gm Protein • 10 gm Carbohydrate • 78 mg Sodium • 14 mg Calcium • 1 gm Fiber

DIABETIC EXCHANGES: 3 Meat • ½ Starch • ½ Fat

CARB CHOICES: ½

Creamed Chicken and Veggies

If your favorite part of the pot pie is the sauce covering the chicken and veggies, then this is the dish for you! Again, if you need to substitute other veggies like green beans for the peas and carrots, it will be okay. But try to use fresh mushrooms, as they really are better in this dish.   ☻   Serves 4 (1 cup)

> 1½ cups diced cooked chicken breast
> 2 cups frozen peas, thawed
> 1½ cups frozen diced or sliced carrots, thawed
> 1 (10¾-ounce) can Healthy Request Cream of Chicken Soup
> ¾ cup water
> ½ cup sliced fresh mushrooms
> 1 teaspoon dried parsley flakes
> ¼ teaspoon black pepper

Spray a pressure cooker container with butter-flavored cooking spray. In prepared container, combine chicken, peas, and carrots. Stir in chicken soup, water, and mushrooms. Add parsley flakes and black pepper. Mix well to combine. Place cover on cooker and bring to LOW pressure over medium heat. Lower heat to stabilize pressure and cook for 3 minutes. Remove from heat, wait for pressure to be released, remove cover, and stir.

HINTS: 1. If you don't have leftovers, purchase a chunk of cooked chicken breast from your local deli.
2. Thaw peas and carrots by rinsing in a colander under hot water for 1 minute.

Each serving equals:

203 Calories • 3 gm Fat • 22 gm Protein • 22 gm Carbohydrate • 425 mg Sodium • 48 mg Calcium • 4 gm Fiber

DIABETIC EXCHANGES: 2 Meat • 1½ Starch/Carbohydrate • 1 Vegetable

CARB CHOICES: 1½

Ultra-Quick Chicken Dinner

I'm promising you fast but I'm also promising you good, so for those nights when you literally have minutes to make dinner before everyone rushes to the table, bookmark this page.

Serves 6 (scant 1 cup)

1 cup uncooked Minute Rice
1 (8-ounce) can cut green beans, undrained
1 medium onion, quartered
½ cup diced green bell pepper
½ cup water
1 (14.5-ounce) can tomatoes, diced in sauce
½ teaspoon chili seasoning
¼ teaspoon black pepper
1 cup diced cooked chicken breast

Spray a pressure cooker container with butter-flavored cooking spray. In prepared container, combine uncooked instant rice, undrained green beans, onion, green pepper, water, and tomatoes. Stir in chili seasoning and black pepper. Place cover on cooker and bring to LOW pressure over medium heat. Lower heat to stabilize pressure and cook for 2 minutes. Remove from heat, wait for pressure to be released, remove cover, and stir. Stir in chicken.

HINT: If you don't have leftovers, purchase a chunk of cooked chicken breast from your local deli.

Each serving equals:

125 Calories • 1 gm Fat • 9 gm Protein • 20 gm Carbohydrate • 475 mg Sodium • 22 mg Calcium • 2 gm Fiber

DIABETIC EXCHANGES: 1 Meat • 1 Starch • 1 Vegetable

CARB CHOICES: 1

Cordon Bleu Dinner Delight

The Cordon Bleu (meaning "blue ribbon") cooking school in Paris is so much more than its best-known dish (chicken with ham and cheese), but this is the recipe that it's become world-famous for. I think this version would win an award, too!

◐ Serves 4 (1¼ cups)

1½ cups diced cooked chicken breast
1 full cup diced Dubuque 97% fat-free ham or any extra-lean ham
1 (10¾-ounce) can Healthy Request Cream of Chicken Soup
1½ cups water

1½ cups frozen peas & carrots, thawed
½ cup chopped onion
1 cup uncooked Minute Rice
1 teaspoon dried parsley flakes
¼ teaspoon black pepper
¾ cup cubed Velveeta 2% Milk processed cheese

Spray a pressure cooker container with butter-flavored cooking spray. In prepared container, combine chicken, ham, chicken soup, and water. Add peas & carrots, onion, uncooked instant rice, parsley flakes, and black pepper. Mix well to combine. Place cover on cooker and bring to LOW pressure over medium heat. Lower heat to stabilize pressure and cook for 4 minutes. Remove from heat, wait for pressure to be released, remove cover, and stir. Add Velveeta cheese. Mix well to combine. Cook over medium heat for 3 to 4 minutes or until cheese melts, stirring often.

HINTS: 1. If you don't have leftovers, purchase a chunk of cooked chicken breast from your local deli.
2. Thaw peas & carrots by rinsing in a colander under hot water for 1 minute.

Each serving equals:

339 Calories • 7 gm Fat • 32 gm Protein • 37 gm Carbohydrate • 1,024 mg Sodium • 161 mg Calcium • 2 gm Fiber

DIABETIC EXCHANGES: 4 Meat • 2 Starch/Carbohydrate • ½ Vegetable

CARB CHOICES: 3

Creole Ham with Rice

This Delta delight is an excellent choice for a weekend supper or even brunch. It's a zesty dish, sure to appeal to folks with hearty appetites who like life just a little spicy. ☺ Serves 4 (1¼ cups)

> 1½ cups diced Dubuque 97% fat-free ham or any extra-lean ham
> 1 cup chopped celery
> 1½ cups coarsely chopped green bell pepper
> ½ cup chopped onion
> ¼ cup reduced-sodium ketchup
> 1 (15-ounce) can diced tomatoes, undrained
> 1 teaspoon dried parsley flakes
> ½ teaspoon dried thyme
> ¼ teaspoon black pepper
> 1 cup uncooked Minute Rice

Spray a pressure cooker container with butter-flavored cooking spray. In prepared container, sauté ham, celery, green pepper, and onion for 3 to 4 minutes. Stir in ketchup, undrained tomatoes, parsley flakes, thyme, and black pepper. Add uncooked instant rice. Mix well to combine. Place cover on cooker and bring to LOW pressure over medium heat. Lower heat to stabilize pressure and cook for 5 minutes. Remove from heat, wait for pressure to be released, remove cover, and stir.

Each serving equals:

214 Calories • 2 gm Fat • 14 gm Protein • 35 gm Carbohydrate • 668 mg Sodium • 46 mg Calcium • 3 gm Fiber

DIABETIC EXCHANGES: 1½ Meat • 1½ Starch • 1½ Vegetable

CARB CHOICES: 2

Country Ham and Corn Casserole

We Iowans joke that we could eat corn at every meal—or at least every day. Our state crop is our pride and palate pleaser, and I've probably created hundreds of corn-based recipes over the years.

☺ Serves 6 (1 cup)

> 2 cups diced Dubuque 97% fat-free ham or any extra-lean ham
> 2 cups frozen whole-kernel corn, thawed
> 2 cups diced unpeeled raw potatoes
> ½ cup chopped celery
> ¼ cup chopped onion
> 1 (10¾-ounce) can Healthy Request Cream of Mushroom Soup
> 1 (2-ounce) jar chopped pimiento, undrained
> ½ cup water
> 1 tablespoon I Can't Believe It's Not Butter! Light Margarine
> ¼ teaspoon black pepper

Spray a pressure cooker container with butter-flavored cooking spray. In prepared container, combine ham, corn, potatoes, celery, and onion. Add mushroom soup, undrained pimiento, water, margarine, and black pepper. Mix well to combine. Place cover on cooker and bring to LOW pressure over medium heat. Lower heat to stabilize pressure and cook for 5 minutes. Remove from heat, wait for pressure to be released, remove cover, and stir.

HINT: Thaw corn by rinsing in a colander under hot water for 1 minute.

Each serving equals:

192 Calories • 4 gm Fat • 12 gm Protein • 27 gm Carbohydrate • 674 mg Sodium • 56 mg Calcium • 3 gm Fiber

DIABETIC EXCHANGES: 1½ Meat • 1½ Starch/Carbohydrate

CARB CHOICES: 2

Cheesy Potato-Ham Scallop

It's a saucy way to enjoy those dynamic partners ham and cheese, coupled with wonderfully filling chunks of potato! When the wind is blowing cold outside, this will warm your insides—and make you grin with pleasure.   ☻   Serves 6 (1 cup)

2 full cups diced Dubuque 97% fat-free ham or any extra-lean ham
3 cups peeled and chopped raw potatoes
1 cup chopped celery
1 cup chopped onion
1 (10¾-ounce) can Healthy Request Cream of Mushroom Soup
¾ cup water
1 teaspoon dried parsley flakes
¼ teaspoon black pepper
¾ cup shredded Kraft reduced-fat Cheddar cheese

Spray a pressure cooker container with butter-flavored cooking spray. In prepared container, combine ham, potatoes, celery, and onion. Add mushroom soup, water, parsley flakes, and black pepper. Mix well to combine. Place cover on cooker and bring to LOW pressure over medium heat. Lower heat to stabilize pressure and cook for 8 minutes. Remove from heat, wait for pressure to be released, remove cover, and stir. Add Cheddar cheese. Mix well to combine.

Each serving equals:

202 Calories • 6 gm Fat • 15 gm Protein • 22 gm Carbohydrate • 659 mg Sodium • 173 mg Calcium • 2 gm Fiber

DIABETIC EXCHANGES: 2 Meat • 1 Starch/Carbohydrate • ½ Vegetable

CARB CHOICES: 1½

Ham and Sweet Surprise

Here's something truly succulent to try with your pressure cooker—a moist and fruity meat-and-potatoes dish that is more than a little out of the ordinary! The nutrients in sweet potatoes are oh-so-good for you, too.   ☺   Serves 4

4 (3-ounce) slices Dubuque 97% fat-free ham or any extra-
    lean ham
4 medium sweet potatoes, halved
1 (8-ounce) can pineapple tidbits, packed in fruit juice,
    undrained
2 tablespoons Splenda Granular
½ teaspoon ground cloves (optional)
½ teaspoon dry mustard

Spray a pressure cooker container with butter-flavored cooking spray. In prepared container, sauté ham slices for 3 to 4 minutes. Arrange sweet potato halves on top of ham slices. Spoon undrained pineapple evenly over potatoes and sprinkle Splenda, cloves, and dry mustard over top. Place cover on cooker and bring to LOW pressure over medium heat. Lower heat to stabilize pressure and cook for 6 minutes. Remove from heat, wait for pressure to be released, and remove cover. When serving, spoon sauce evenly over ham and sweet potato slices.

HINTS: 1. A 3-ounce slice of ham is about ⅓ inch thick.
       2. If you can't find pineapple tidbits, use chunk pineapple
          and coarsely chop.

Each serving equals:

214 Calories • 2 gm Fat • 16 gm Protein • 33 gm Carbohydrate • 741 mg Sodium •
47 mg Calcium • 4 gm Fiber

DIABETIC EXCHANGES: 2 Meat • 2 Starch • ½ Fruit

CARB CHOICES: 2½

Mushroom-Laced Pork Tenders

I love coming up with new and exciting ways to cook pork tenders. It's a superbly satisfying cut of meat that also delivers good nutrition and less fat. Make sure you choose mushrooms that don't have dark spots and are tightly closed, not spongy.   ☻   Serves 4

6 tablespoons all-purpose flour☆
2 teaspoons dried parsley flakes
¼ teaspoon black pepper
1 tablespoon prepared yellow mustard
4 (4-ounce) lean pork tenderloins
1 tablespoon vegetable oil
1 (10¾-ounce) can Healthy Request Cream of Mushroom
    Soup
½ cup sliced fresh mushrooms
1 cup water

In a shallow saucer, combine 3 tablespoons flour, parsley flakes, and black pepper. Evenly spread ¼ teaspoon mustard on each side of tenderloins. Coat tenderloins on each side in flour mixture. Spray a pressure cooker container with butter-flavored cooking spray. Sprinkle vegetable oil in bottom of cooker container. Arrange coated tenderloins evenly in prepared container and brown for 3 minutes on each side. In a small bowl, combine mushroom soup, mushrooms, water, and any remaining flour mixture. Evenly pour mixture over tenderloins. Place cover on cooker and bring to LOW pressure over medium heat. Lower heat to stabilize pressure and cook for 10 minutes. Remove from heat, wait for pressure to be released, and remove cover. Remove tenderloins from cooker. Drain off ½ cup liquid. In a covered jar, combine liquid and remaining 3 tablespoons flour. Shake well to blend. Add flour mixture to cooker. Cook over medium heat for 2 to 3 minutes or until mixture is thickened, stirring constantly. For each serving, place 1 tenderloin on a plate and spoon ½ cup sauce mixture over top.

Each serving equals:

245 Calories • 9 gm Fat • 26 gm Protein • 15 gm Carbohydrate • 390 mg Sodium • 72 mg Calcium • 1 gm Fiber

DIABETIC EXCHANGES: 3 Meat • 1 Starch/Carbohydrate • 1 Fat

CARB CHOICES: 1

Oriental Pork

Asian menus feature all kinds of pork dishes, so I was inspired to invent my own tangy approach to this meat, which can be cooked so many different ways. It's so good, you'll want to serve it often, so pick up a package of the Splenda Brown Sugar Blend. You'll be glad you did! ❂ Serves 4

> 4 (4-ounce) lean pork tenderloins
> ½ cup chopped onion
> ¼ cup chili sauce
> 1 cube Knorr Vegetable Bouillon
> 2 cups water
> 2 tablespoons reduced-sodium soy sauce
> 1 teaspoon dried minced garlic
> 1 tablespoon Splenda Brown Sugar Blend
> 4 tablespoons all-purpose flour

Spray a pressure cooker container with olive oil–flavored cooking spray. In prepared container, sauté tenderloins for 3 minutes on each side. In a small bowl, combine onion, chili sauce, dry vegetable bouillon, water, soy sauce, garlic, and Splenda. Evenly pour mixture over tenderloins. Place cover on cooker and bring to LOW pressure over medium heat. Lower heat to stabilize pressure and cook for 12 minutes. Remove from heat, wait for pressure to be released, remove cover, and stir. Remove tenderloins from cooker. Drain off ¾ cup liquid. In a covered jar, combine liquid and flour. Shake well to blend. Add flour mixture to cooker. Cook over medium heat for 2 to 3 minutes or until mixture is thickened, stirring constantly. For each serving, place 1 tenderloin on a plate and spoon about ¾ cup sauce mixture over top.

Each serving equals:

171 Calories • 3 gm Fat • 20 gm Protein • 16 gm Carbohydrate • 323 mg Sodium • 18 mg Calcium • 0 gm Fiber

DIABETIC EXCHANGES: 3 Meat • 1 Starch/Carbohydrate

CARB CHOICES: 1

Pork Supper Pot

I love the one-pot-style meals you can prepare in today's pressure cookers, and this one is especially easy. You'll see that I do the meat first, then add the rest of the veggies. Don't forget to remove the bay leaf—it's not good for you. ☻ Serves 6 (1 cup)

> 16 ounces lean pork tenderloin, cut into bite-size pieces
> 1 cup chopped onion
> 1½ cups sliced celery
> 1 cup water
> 2 cups diced unpeeled potatoes
> 1½ cups sliced carrots
> 1 cup frozen peas, thawed
> ¼ teaspoon black pepper
> 1 bay leaf

Spray a pressure cooker container with butter-flavored cooking spray. In prepared container, sauté pork pieces, onion, and celery for 5 minutes. Add water, potatoes, carrots, peas, black pepper, and bay leaf. Mix well to combine. Place cover on cooker and bring to LOW pressure over medium heat. Lower heat to stabilize pressure and cook for 10 minutes. Remove from heat, wait for pressure to be released, remove cover, and stir. Remove bay leaf before serving.

HINT: Thaw peas by rinsing in a colander under hot water for 1 minute.

Each serving equals:

150 Calories • 2 gm Fat • 15 gm Protein • 18 gm Carbohydrate • 105 mg Sodium • 42 mg Calcium • 3 gm Fiber

DIABETIC EXCHANGES: 2 Meat • 1 Vegetable • ½ Starch

CARB CHOICES: 1

German Dinner Pot

Here's a perfect Oktoberfest meal—but you don't need a holiday to enjoy it. Its flavor is unique, and you'll surely leave the table with a satisfied tummy.   ❂   Serves 4 (1½ cups)

> *16 ounces lean pork tenderloin, cut into bite-size pieces*
> *¾ cup chopped onion*
> *1 (8-ounce) can Hunt's Tomato Sauce*
> *1 cup water*
> *1 (14½-ounce) can Frank's Bavarian-style sauerkraut,*
> *   drained*
> *1 teaspoon dried parsley flakes*
> *¼ teaspoon black pepper*
> *1 cup uncooked Minute Rice*

Spray a pressure cooker container with butter-flavored cooking spray. In prepared container, sauté pork pieces, and onion for 3 to 4 minutes. Stir in tomato sauce, water, sauerkraut, parsley flakes, and black pepper. Add uncooked instant rice. Mix well to combine. Place cover on cooker and bring to LOW pressure over medium heat. Lower heat to stabilize pressure and cook for 6 minutes. Remove from heat, wait for pressure to be released, remove cover, and stir.

HINT: If you can't find Bavarian-style sauerkraut, use regular sauerkraut, ½ teaspoon caraway seeds, and 1 teaspoon Brown Sugar Twin.

Each serving equals:

274 Calories • 6 gm Fat • 26 gm Protein • 29 gm Carbohydrate • 355 mg Sodium • 24 mg Calcium • 2 gm Fiber

DIABETIC EXCHANGES: 3 Meat • 2 Vegetable • 1 Starch

CARB CHOICES: 2

Mom's Corned Beef and Cabbage

The traditional version of this Irish classic can take hours, even days, to prepare. Not anymore! St. Paddy's Day comes but once a year, and that's not often enough to enjoy this traditional treat.

● Serves 4 (1 cup)

> 3 cups coarsely chopped cabbage
> 2 cups peeled and diced raw potatoes
> 1 cup fresh or frozen sliced carrots, thawed
> ½ cup chopped onion
> 3 (2.5-ounce) packages Carl Buddig lean corned beef,
>   shredded
> 1 (10¾-ounce) can Healthy Request Cream of Mushroom
>   Soup
> ¼ cup water

Spray a pressure cooker container with butter-flavored cooking spray. In prepared container, combine cabbage, potatoes, carrots, and onion. Stir in corned beef. Add mushroom soup and water. Mix well to combine. Place cover on cooker and bring to LOW pressure over medium heat. Lower heat to stabilize pressure and cook for 6 minutes. Remove from heat, wait for pressure to be released, remove cover, and stir.

HINT: Thaw carrots by rinsing in a colander under hot water for 1 minute.

Each serving equals:

205 Calories • 5 gm Fat • 13 gm Protein • 27 gm Carbohydrate •
1,035 mg Sodium • 111 mg Calcium • 4 gm Fiber

DIABETIC EXCHANGES: 2 Meat • 1½ Starch/Carbohydrate • 1½ Vegetable

CARB CHOICES: 2

Aaron's Macaroni and Hot Dogs ❄

I once said to my grandson Aaron, "Should we have hot dogs for lunch, or mac and cheese?" He gave me the sweetest smile and said, "Both!" Inspired, I created this dish that celebrates both his special favorites.   ◐   Serves 4 (1 cup)

1 cup uncooked elbow macaroni
1 cup frozen green beans, thawed
4 ounces Oscar Mayer or Healthy Choice reduced-fat
    frankfurters, diced
1 (10¾-ounce) can Healthy Request Cream of Mushroom
    Soup
1¼ cups water
1½ cups cubed Velveeta 2% Milk processed cheese

Spray a pressure cooker container with butter-flavored cooking spray. In prepared container, combine uncooked macaroni, green beans, frankfurters, mushroom soup, and water. Place cover on cooker and bring to LOW pressure over medium heat. Lower heat to stabilize pressure and cook for 4 minutes. Remove from heat, wait for pressure to be released, remove cover, and stir. Add Velveeta cheese. Mix well to combine. Cook over medium heat for 3 to 4 minutes or until cheese melts, stirring often.

HINT: Thaw green beans by rinsing in a colander under hot water
    for 1 minute.

Each serving equals:

267 Calories • 7 gm Fat • 16 gm Protein • 35 gm Carbohydrate •
1,251 mg Sodium • 324 mg Calcium • 2 gm Fiber

DIABETIC EXCHANGES: 2 Meat • 2 Starch/Carbohydrate • ½ Vegetable

CARB CHOICES: 2

Josh's Speedy Spaghetti

Cooking for kids can be an endless job for busy moms, but cooking *with* kids often provides great ideas for family-pleasing meals. Josh is a boy in a hurry, always busy with some new project. I hope he thinks this dish is ready soon enough! ☻ Serves 6 (1 cup)

> 1 (15-ounce) can diced tomatoes, undrained
> 1½ cups reduced-sodium tomato juice
> 1 cup water
> 1 (10¾-ounce) can Healthy Request Tomato Soup
> 1½ teaspoons Italian seasoning
> 2 cups broken uncooked spaghetti
> 2 tablespoons Kraft Reduced Fat Parmesan Style Grated
>   Topping

Spray a pressure cooker container with olive oil–flavored cooking spray. In prepared container, combine undrained tomatoes, tomato juice, water, tomato soup, and Italian seasoning. Add uncooked spaghetti. Mix well to combine. Place cover on cooker and bring to LOW pressure over medium heat. Lower heat to stabilize pressure and cook for 5 minutes. Remove from heat, wait for pressure to be released, remove cover, and stir. When serving, sprinkle 1 teaspoon Parmesan cheese over each dish.

Each serving equals:

193 Calories • 1 gm Fat • 6 gm Protein • 40 gm Carbohydrate • 402 mg Sodium • 27 mg Calcium • 3 gm Fiber

DIABETIC EXCHANGES: 2 Starch/Carbohydrate • 1 Vegetable

CARB CHOICES: 2½

A Terrific Taste
of This and That

Whenever I look through a new cookbook (or, for that matter, a nice old vintage one from my collection), I love to turn past the usual sections of appetizers and main dishes and head for the recipes that defy classification—the ones that are beloved of the author but that don't fit into the other categories. That's where I know I'll find the "fun stuff": festive sauces and luscious ideas for brunch, among others.

What can you look forward to trying from this section? Pressure cookers make canning a breeze, so if you've never done that before, you have so much to look forward to! You've got a treat ahead of you with my Fruit Compote, *a whole new way to enjoy nature's sweet bounty. The* Spiced Apples *are wonderful, as are the* Citrus Pudding *and the* Rice Pudding Extraordinaire. *If you love beans, I hope you'll try* Duke's Red Beans. *I'm also proud of my* Piccadilly Salsa *and, for you "heat" lovers,* Not for Sissies Salsa. *Enjoy!*

Spiced Apples

Apples are born sweet, and some might say that they need nothing else to be perfectly delicious. But—and I speak for myself here—I think that they are even more mouthwatering when cooked and spiced in just this way. I like them on my cereal. Mmm-mm!

● Serves 6 (⅔ cup)

> 5 cups (5 medium) cored and peeled cooking apples, cut in
> ½-inch slices
> 1 cup unsweetened orange juice
> ¾ cup Splenda Granular
> 1 cup Brown Sugar Twin
> 2 teaspoons apple pie spice
> ½ teaspoon rum extract
> 2 tablespoons cornstarch
> ½ cup water

Spray a pressure cooker container with butter-flavored cooking spray. In prepared container, combine apples, orange juice, Splenda, Brown Sugar Twin, apple pie spice, and rum extract. Place cover on cooker and bring to LOW pressure over medium heat. Lower heat to stabilize pressure and cook for 4 minutes. Remove from heat, wait for pressure to be released, remove cover, and stir. In a covered jar, combine cornstarch and water. Shake well to blend. Stir cornstarch mixture into apple mixture. Cook over medium heat for 3 to 4 minutes, stirring often.

HINT: Good served over pound cake, waffles, French toast, or ice cream.

Each serving equals:

100 Calories • 0 gm Fat • 0 gm Protein • 25 gm Carbohydrate • 1 mg Sodium • 11 mg Calcium • 2 gm Fiber

DIABETIC EXCHANGES: 1½ Fruit

CARB CHOICES: 1½

Fruit Compote

Here's another fantastic use for the pressure cooker—to prepare an old-fashioned fruit compote that used to require hours of stirring over a hot stove. If you can't find frozen apricots, feel free to substitute another fruit. The finished dish will differ but should still be luscious. (Try cherries for a colorful twist!)

❂ Serves 6 (½ cup)

> 1 (8-ounce) package frozen apricots, thawed
> 1 (8-ounce) package frozen peaches, thawed
> 1 (8-ounce) can crushed pineapple, undrained
> ¾ cup water
> ½ cup Splenda Granular
> 1 teaspoon ground cinnamon
> ¼ teaspoon ground nutmeg
> 1 tablespoon cold water
> 1 tablespoon cornstarch

Spray a pressure cooker container with butter-flavored cooking spray. In prepared container, combine apricots, peaches, undrained pineapple, and water. Stir in Splenda, cinnamon, and nutmeg. Place cover on cooker and bring to LOW pressure over medium heat. Lower heat to stabilize pressure and cook for 5 minutes. Remove from heat, wait for pressure to be released, remove cover, and stir. In a covered jar, combine cold water and cornstarch. Shake well to blend. Stir cornstarch mixture into fruit mixture. Cook over medium heat for 1 to 2 minutes or until mixture is thickened, stirring constantly.

HINT: Good served over pound cake, over ice cream, or as a light dessert.

Each serving equals:

80 Calories • 0 gm Fat • 0 gm Protein • 20 gm Carbohydrate • 2 mg Sodium • 14 mg Calcium • 1 gm Fiber

DIABETIC EXCHANGES: 1 Fruit

CARB CHOICES: 1

Citrus Pudding

It's always fun to find new ways to use one of my favorite spring delights, rhubarb. This recipe works just fine with frozen, too, so don't feel you have to wait for warmer months to savor it.

◐ Serves 4 (¾ cup)

> 1 pound fresh or frozen rhubarb, cut in 1-inch pieces
> ½ cup + 2 tablespoons water☆
> 1 cup unsweetened orange juice
> ¾ cup Splenda Granular
> 1 tablespoon all-purpose flour

In a pressure cooker container, combine rhubarb, ½ cup water, orange juice, and Splenda. Place cover on cooker and bring to LOW pressure over medium heat. Lower heat to stabilize pressure and cook for 2 minutes. Remove from heat, wait for pressure to be released, remove cover, and stir. In a covered jar, combine flour and remaining 2 tablespoons water. Shake well to blend. Stir flour mixture into rhubarb mixture. Simmer for 2 minutes or until mixture comes to a boil and starts to thicken, stirring constantly.

Each serving equals:

72 Calories • 0 gm Fat • 1 gm Protein • 17 gm Carbohydrate • 5 mg Sodium • 104 mg Calcium • 2 gm Fiber

DIABETIC EXCHANGES: 1 Fruit

CARB CHOICES: 1

Rice Pudding Extraordinaire

Every truck stop across the country, and probably most of the diners you pass, serves rice pudding—and some of it is very tasty. But this version is worth driving out of your way for, and you don't have to go farther than your own kitchen!　　🌑　Serves 6 (½ cup)

> 2 tablespoons I Can't Believe It's Not Butter! Light
>   Margarine
> 2 cups fat-free milk
> 1 cup Land O Lakes Fat Free Half & Half
> 1 cup uncooked long-grain rice
> ⅓ cup Splenda Granular
> 1 teaspoon vanilla extract
> Ground cinnamon

Spray a pressure cooker container with butter-flavored cooking spray. In prepared container, melt margarine. Add milk and half & half. Mix well to combine. Bring to a boil. Stir in uncooked rice. Place cover on cooker and bring to LOW pressure over medium heat. Lower heat to stabilize pressure and cook for 10 minutes. Remove from heat, wait for pressure to be released, remove cover, and stir. Stir in Splenda and vanilla extract. When serving, sprinkle cinnamon over each.

Each serving equals:

130 Calories • 2 gm Fat • 5 gm Protein • 23 gm Carbohydrate • 130 mg Sodium • 156 mg Calcium • 0 gm Fiber

DIABETIC EXCHANGES: 1½ Starch/Carbohydrate

CARB CHOICES: 1½

Harvest-Time Oatmeal

Tired of the same hot cereal, day after chilly winter day? Or worse, have you gotten into the habit of using those instant packets? Here's a warm and wonderful breakfast treat that will change the way you view this morning staple!   ☾   Serves 6 (½ cup)

> 1 cup water
> ¼ cup fat-free milk
> 2 tablespoons + 2 teaspoons I Can't Believe It's Not Butter! Light Margarine
> ½ teaspoon apple pie spice
> 1½ cups (3 small) cored, peeled, and chopped cooking apples
> ½ cup chopped dried apricots
> ½ cup Land O Lakes Fat Free Half & Half
> ⅓ cup Log Cabin Sugar Free Maple Syrup
> 1 cup quick oats
> ¼ cup chopped pecans

Spray a pressure cooker container with butter-flavored cooking spray. In prepared container, combine water, milk, margarine, and apple pie spice. Stir in apples and apricots. Place cover on cooker and bring to LOW pressure over medium heat. Lower heat to stabilize pressure and cook for 2 minutes. Remove from heat, wait for pressure to be released, remove cover, and stir. Add half & half, maple syrup, oats, and pecans. Mix well to combine. Let set for 2 to 3 minutes before serving.

Each serving equals:

183 Calories • 7 gm Fat • 4 gm Protein • 26 gm Carbohydrate • 110 mg Sodium • 61 mg Calcium • 4 gm Fiber

DIABETIC EXCHANGES: 1 Starch • 1 Fruit • 1 Fat

CARB CHOICES: 2

Spicy Cream of Wheat with Walnuts

Sometimes all it takes to make the familiar special is a touch of spice and a sprinkling of nuts. If you're a Cream of Wheat lover, it's time to light a new fire under that passion.

◉ Serves 4 (¾ cup)

> 3 cups boiling water
> ½ cup Cream of Wheat
> ½ teaspoon table salt
> 1½ teaspoons ground cinnamon
> 2 tablespoons chopped walnuts

Spray a pressure cooker container with butter-flavored cooking spray. In prepared container, combine water and Cream of Wheat. Add salt and cinnamon. Mix well to combine. Place cover on cooker and bring to LOW pressure over medium heat. Lower heat to stabilize pressure and cook for 2 minutes. Remove from heat, wait for pressure to be released, remove cover, and stir. Stir in walnuts.

Each serving equals:

95 Calories • 3 gm Fat • 3 gm Protein • 14 gm Carbohydrate • 293 mg Sodium • 19 mg Calcium • 3 gm Fiber

DIABETIC EXCHANGES: 1 Starch • ½ Fat

CARB CHOICES: 1

Anytime Butter Beans

This bean dish is so tasty, your kids may ask to snack on it after school instead of salty chips or other junk food.

🕒 Serves 6 (⅔ cup)

> 1 cup diced Dubuque 97% fat-free ham or any extra-lean ham
> ½ cup diced onion
> 1 stalk celery, diced
> 1 cup diced carrots
> 1 (14-ounce) can Swanson Lower Sodium Fat Free Chicken Broth
> 1 tablespoon dried parsley flakes
> ¼ teaspoon black pepper
> 1 (15-ounce) can butter beans, rinsed and drained

Spray a pressure cooker container with butter-flavored cooking spray. In prepared container, sauté ham pieces, onion, and celery for 4 to 5 minutes. Add carrots, chicken broth, parsley flakes, and black pepper. Mix well to combine. Place cover on cooker and bring to LOW pressure over medium heat. Lower heat to stabilize pressure and cook for 4 minutes. Remove from heat, wait for pressure to be released, remove cover, and stir. Add butter beans. Mix well to combine. Cook over medium heat for 2 to 3 minutes.

Each serving equals:

85 Calories • 1 gm Fat • 8 gm Protein • 11 gm Carbohydrate • 403 mg Sodium • 38 mg Calcium • 3 gm Fiber

DIABETIC EXCHANGES: 1 Meat • ½ Starch • ½ Vegetable

CARB CHOICES: 1

Delicious Black Beans

For your next party, leave the commercial dips at the store and stir up your own bowl of beguiling black beans! Try this with blue corn chips or make your own chips from flavored tortillas.

○ Serves 6 (full 1 cup)

> 2 cups dried black beans
> 1 cup chopped onion
> 1 teaspoon dried minced garlic
> ½ cup chopped green bell pepper
> 1 (14-ounce) can Swanson Lower Sodium Fat Free Beef
>   Broth
> ½ cup spicy salsa

In a large bowl, soak black beans in hot water overnight or for at least 1 hour. Drain and rinse well. Spray a pressure cooker container with butter-flavored cooking spray. In prepared container, sauté onion for 2 to 3 minutes. Add beans, garlic, green pepper, and beef broth. Mix well to combine. Place cover on cooker and bring to LOW pressure over medium heat. Lower heat to stabilize pressure and cook for 12 minutes. Remove from heat, wait for pressure to be released, remove cover, and stir. Stir in salsa.

HINT: If you like your salsa less spicy, use mild or medium.

Each serving equals:

180 Calories • 0 gm Fat • 10 gm Protein • 34 gm Carbohydrate • 285 mg Sodium • 7 mg Calcium • 4 gm Fiber

DIABETIC EXCHANGES: 1½ Starch • 1 Meat • 1 Vegetable

CARB CHOICES: 2

Duke's Red Beans

No, I don't actually serve this to our wonderful and amazing dog, Duke, but he must know it's good because he wouldn't leave the kitchen while we were testing the recipe! So, I named it after him. I love you, Duke! ☺ Serves 8 (1 cup)

> 2 cups dried red beans
> 1 cup chopped onion
> 2 tablespoons dried minced garlic
> 2 carrots, finely chopped
> 2 stalks celery, finely chopped
> 1 (15-ounce) can diced tomatoes, undrained
> 1 cup diced Dubuque 97% fat-free ham or any extra-lean
>   ham
> 2 cups water
> ¼ teaspoon black pepper
> 2 teaspoons chili seasoning

In a large bowl, soak red beans in hot water overnight or for at least 1 hour. Drain and rinse well. Spray a pressure cooker container with butter-flavored cooking spray. In prepared container, sauté onion and garlic for 2 to 3 minutes. Add beans, carrots, celery, undrained tomatoes, ham, water, and black pepper. Mix well to combine. Place cover on cooker and bring to LOW pressure over medium heat. Lower heat to stabilize pressure and cook for 25 minutes. Remove from heat, wait for pressure to be released, remove cover, and stir. Stir in chili seasoning.

HINT: Good served over rice.

Each serving equals:

217 Calories • 1 gm Fat • 15 gm Protein • 37 gm Carbohydrate • 325 mg Sodium • 95 mg Calcium • 5 gm Fiber

DIABETIC EXCHANGES: 2 Meat • 2 Starch • 1 Vegetable

CARB CHOICES: 2

Boston-Style Peas

This is the way they like their black-eyed peas up North, which is very different from how they prefer 'em down South. I like knowing that even while I'm staying at Timber Ridge Farm, I can travel anywhere I like through the magic of regional foods!

☻ Serves 6 (1 cup)

2 cups dried black-eyed peas
2 cups hot water
¼ cup chopped onion
1 tablespoon dry mustard
½ teaspoon table salt
¼ teaspoon black pepper
2 ¼ cups water
⅓ cup Log Cabin Sugar Free Maple Syrup
2 tablespoons Oscar Mayer or Hormel Real Bacon Bits

In a large bowl, soak black-eyed peas in hot water overnight or for at least 1 hour. Drain and rinse well. Spray a pressure cooker container with butter-flavored cooking spray. In prepared container, sauté onion for 3 to 4 minutes. Add peas, dry mustard, salt, black pepper, and water. Mix well to combine. Place cover on cooker and bring to LOW pressure over medium heat. Lower heat to stabilize pressure and cook for 30 minutes. Remove from heat, wait for pressure to be released, remove cover, and stir. Stir in maple syrup and bacon bits.

Each serving equals:

209 Calories • 1 gm Fat • 14 gm Protein • 36 gm Carbohydrate • 308 mg Sodium • 63 mg Calcium • 6 gm Fiber

DIABETIC EXCHANGES: 2 Starch • 1½ Meat

CARB CHOICES: 2

Cranapple Sauce

Tart and rosy, cranberries are one of those fruits that can't be enjoyed on their own without some cooking and sweetening. Partnered with some apples, though, and bathed in juice, they form the basis for a splendid sauce. ☺ Serves 8 (⅔ cup)

> 3 pounds (8 medium) cored, peeled, and quartered Red
>   Delicious apples
> 1½ cups fresh or frozen cranberries
> 1 teaspoon ground cinnamon
> 1 cup unsweetened apple juice
> ¼ cup Splenda Granular

Spray a pressure cooker container with butter-flavored cooking spray. In prepared container, combine apples, cranberries, cinnamon, apple juice, and Splenda. Place cover on cooker and bring to LOW pressure over medium heat. Lower heat to stabilize pressure and cook for 10 minutes. Remove from heat, wait for pressure to be released, remove cover, and stir. Puree apple mixture with a handheld potato masher or process with a hand blender in the pressure cooker container. Add additional Splenda and cinnamon, if desired. Refrigerate until cool.

Each serving equals:

120 Calories • 0 gm Fat • 0 gm Protein • 30 gm Carbohydrate • 3 mg Sodium • 17 mg Calcium • 5 gm Fiber

DIABETIC EXCHANGES: 2 Fruit

CARB CHOICES: 1½

Piccadilly Salsa

It's one of the liveliest and most fun parts of London—Piccadilly Circus, where the streets are filled with people at all hours of the day and night! When I was naming this lively recipe, I thought "Piccadilly Salsa"—the salsa that is equally as alive as its namesake.

☺ Serves 16 (¼ cup)

2 large ripe tomatoes, each peeled and cut into 6 wedges
1 large cucumber, seeds removed and finely chopped
½ cup finely chopped onion
1 tablespoon fresh parsley or 1 teaspoon dried parsley flakes
3 tablespoons Splenda Granular

Spray a pressure cooker container with butter-flavored cooking spray. In prepared container, combine tomatoes, cucumber, onion, parsley, and Splenda. Place cover on cooker and bring to LOW pressure over medium heat. Lower heat to stabilize pressure and cook for 5 minutes. Remove from heat, wait for pressure to be released, remove cover, and stir. Store in refrigerator up to 2 weeks.

Each serving equals:

8 Calories • 0 gm Fat • 0 gm Protein • 2 gm Carbohydrate • 1 mg Sodium • 6 mg Calcium • 0 gm Fiber

DIABETIC EXCHANGES: 1 Free Food

CARB CHOICES: 0

Not for Sissies Salsa

If you love things HOT, HOT, HOT, then come on over and dig your favorite chips into this five-alarm salsa! Cliff loved it; my tongue burned after one tiny taste. You hotties out there—you know who you are—enjoy! ☻ Serves 20 (¼ cup)

9 cups peeled and chopped fresh tomatoes
1½ cups chopped onion
½ cup finely chopped celery
1 cup chopped green bell pepper
3 jalapeño peppers, seeds removed and chopped
3 large cloves of garlic
¼ cup Splenda Granular

Spray a pressure cooker container with olive oil–flavored cooking spray. In prepared container, combine tomatoes, onion, celery, green pepper, and jalapeño peppers. Add garlic and Splenda. Mix well to combine. Place cover on cooker and bring to LOW pressure over medium heat. Lower heat to stabilize pressure and cook for 5 minutes. Remove from heat, wait for pressure to be released, remove cover, and stir. Store in refrigerator up to 2 weeks or in freezer up to 3 months.

Each serving equals:

24 Calories • 0 gm Fat • 1 gm Protein • 5 gm Carbohydrate • 7 mg Sodium • 13 mg Calcium • 1 gm Fiber

DIABETIC EXCHANGES: 1 Free Food

CARB CHOICES: 0

Zucchini Marinara Sauce

When the zucchini harvest threatens to overwhelm you, quick—make lots of tomato sauce and share it with everyone you love! It's perfect over pasta, very good on veggies, and great on grilled chicken and fish.　　◐　Serves 4 (¾ cup)

> 4 cups sliced unpeeled zucchini
> ½ cup chopped onion
> 1 (8-ounce) can Hunt's Tomato Sauce
> ½ cup reduced-sodium tomato juice
> 2 tablespoons Kraft Fat Free Italian Dressing
> 1 teaspoon Splenda Granular
> 1 teaspoon dried minced garlic
> ¼ teaspoon black pepper

Spray a pressure cooker container with olive oil–flavored cooking spray. In prepared container, combine zucchini, onion, tomato sauce, tomato juice, and Italian dressing. Add Splenda, garlic, and black pepper. Mix well to combine. Place cover on cooker and bring to LOW pressure over medium heat. Lower heat to stabilize pressure and cook for 5 minutes. Remove from heat, wait for pressure to be released, remove cover, and stir.

Each serving equals:

60 Calories • 0 gm Fat • 2 gm Protein • 13 gm Carbohydrate • 449 mg Sodium • 36 mg Calcium • 2 gm Fiber

DIABETIC EXCHANGES: 2 Vegetable

CARB CHOICES: 1

Italian Tomato Wedges

Calling all canners out there across America! Buy the ripest, reddest, most beautiful tomatoes you can find (or pick them from your own plants) and get to work. You'll feast on this recipe all winter long.   ☉   Makes 5 pints

> 5 pounds tomatoes, peeled and quartered
> ½ pound onions, sliced thin
> 2 green bell peppers, sliced into ¼ inch strips
> 5 teaspoons Italian seasoning
> 1¼ teaspoons parsley
> 1 tablespoon vinegar

In a large saucepan, combine tomatoes, onions, and green peppers. Bring to a boil over medium heat and cook for 5 minutes. Carefully ladle hot mixture into 5 hot standard pint jars made for home canning. Add 1 teaspoon Italian seasoning and ¼ teaspoon parsley to each jar. Cover with boiling water, leaving 1 inch of headspace. Wipe rim of jars clean so no seeds, pulp, or liquid prevents a good seal. Seal with new metal band and lids according to manufacturer's instructions. Place rack in cooker. Pour in 2 quarts of hot water. Add 1 tablespoon vinegar to help prevent water stains in cooker and on jars. Place jars on rack in pressure cooker container. Place cover on cooker and bring to LOW pressure over medium heat. Lower heat to stabilize pressure and cook for 15 minutes. Remove from heat and wait for pressure to be released, about 25 to 30 minutes, then remove cover. Using a jar lifter, remove jars from cooker and set on a cooling rack. Allow jars to cool completely. Wipe jars with a damp cloth. Dry and label with contents and date. Store in a cool, dry place.

Each ½ cup serving equals:

28 Calories • 0 gm Fat • 1 gm Protein • 6 gm Carbohydrate • 6 mg Sodium • 16 mg Calcium • 2 gm Fiber

DIABETIC EXCHANGES: 1 Vegetable

CARB CHOICES: ½

Connie's Canned Peaches

If you've never canned your own peaches, make this the year you do, with this version of Connie's best peach canning recipe! Peaches have a short season in the summer, and while commercial canned peaches are okay, they don't hold a candle to the home-canned "real thing!"   ☻   Serves 16 (½ cup)

  12 medium-size fresh ripe peaches
  2 cups water
  1 cup Splenda Granular
  1 tablespoon vinegar

Dip peaches into boiling water, then into cold water. Slip off skins. Cut in half and remove pits. Place in water to which lemon juice or ascorbic acid has been added to keep fruit from darkening before it is packed. Meanwhile, in a large saucepan, prepare syrup by combining 2 cups water and Splenda. Bring to a boil. Drain peaches and pack into 4 hot standard pint jars made for home canning. Carefully ladle boiling syrup over peaches, leaving a ½-inch headspace. Wipe rim of jars clean so no seeds, pulp, or liquid prevent a good seal. Seal with new metal band and lids according to manufacturer's instructions. Place rack in cooker. Pour in 2 quarts of hot water. Add 1 tablespoon vinegar to help prevent water stains in cooker and on jars. Place jars on rack in pressure cooker container. Place cover on cooker and bring to LOW pressure over medium heat. Lower heat to stabilize pressure and cook for 10 minutes. Remove from heat and wait for pressure to be released, about 25 to 30 minutes, then remove cover. Using a jar lifter, remove jars from cooker and set on a cooling rack. Allow jars to cool completely. Wipe jars with a damp cloth. Dry and label with contents and date. Store in cool, dry place.

Each serving equals:

32 Calories • 0 gm Fat • 0 gm Protein • 8 gm Carbohydrate • 0 mg Sodium • 4 mg Calcium • 1 gm Fiber

DIABETIC EXCHANGES: ½ Fruit

CARB CHOICES: ½

Cheryl's Canned Corn

Cheryl helps me test my recipes, and this is her special way of preparing canned corn. Once you taste the fantastic result, you'll regret only that you don't have more shelves to stack the jars on!

◗ Serves 16 (½ cup)

> 15 medium-size ears sweet corn
> 4 cups boiling water
> 1 tablespoon vinegar

Remove husks from corn and cut kernels from cob. Pack kernels loosely into 4 hot standard pint jars made for home canning. Pour boiling water over corn, leaving a 1-inch headspace. Wipe rim of jars clean so no seeds, pulp, or liquid prevents a good seal. Seal with new metal band and lids according to manufacturer's instructions. Place rack in cooker. Pour in 2 quarts of hot water. Add 1 tablespoon vinegar to help prevent water stains in cooker and on jars. Place jars on rack in pressure cooker container. Place cover on cooker and bring to LOW pressure over medium heat. Lower heat to stabilize pressure and cook for 55 minutes. Remove from heat and wait for pressure to be released, about 25 to 30 minutes, then remove cover. Using a jar lifter, remove jars from cooker and set on a cooling rack. Allow jars to cool completely. Wipe jars with a damp cloth. Dry and label with contents and date. Store in cool, dry place.

Each serving equals:

81 Calories • 1 gm Fat • 2 gm Protein • 16 gm Carbohydrate • 12 mg Sodium • 1 mg Calcium • 2 gm Fiber

---

DIABETIC EXCHANGES: 1 Starch

CARB CHOICES: 1

Menus to Help You "Handle the Pressure"

Your pressure cooker is better than a therapist when you're feeling like a juggler who's about to drop all her whirling plates! With the help of this handy appliance, dishes that could normally take hours to prepare are instead ready in minutes. Here are some fun ways to shine a spotlight on this unsung kitchen superstar!

"Almost-Too-Cold-to-Cook" Winter Night Delight

Momma Mia Minestrone

Sweet Potatoes Supreme

Chicken Fricassee

Fruit Compote

"It's April Already" Tax Time Buffet

Cream of Potato and Pea Soup

Asparagus in Dijon Butter

Chicken Veronique

Rice Pudding Extraordinaire

"Back to School" Labor Day Supper

Southwest Corn and Ham Chowder

Summer Garden Special

Shrimp Creole

Connie's Canned Peaches (over fat-free and sugar-free ice cream!)

"Carpool Time" Family Chowdown

Cheesy Tater Chowder

Tangy Red Cabbage

Chicken-Macaroni Pot Pie

Citrus Pudding

"I'm on a Deadline" Last-Minute Dinner

Spiced Acorn Squash

Cheesy Creamed Corn

Cliff's Sloppy Joes

Duke's Red Beans

"Five Days Until Christmas" Speedy Sunday Brunch

Neapolitan Tomato Bisque

Nutty Green Beans

Pizza Pot Casserole

Spiced Apples

Making Healthy Exchanges Work for You

Y ou're ready now to begin a wonderful journey to better health. In the preceding pages, you've discovered the remarkable variety of good food available to you when you begin eating the Healthy Exchanges way. You've stocked your pantry and learned many of my food preparation "secrets," which will point you on the way to delicious success.

But before I let you go, I'd like to share a few tips that I've learned while traveling toward healthier eating habits. It took me a long time to learn how to eat *smarter*. In fact, I'm still working on it, but I am getting better. For years I could *inhale* a five-course meal in five minutes flat—and still make room for a second helping of dessert!

Now I follow certain signposts on the road that help me stay on the right path. I hope these ideas will help point you in the right direction as well.

1. **Eat slowly** so your brain has time to catch up with your tummy. Cut and chew each bite slowly. Try putting your fork down between bites. Stop eating as soon as you feel full. Crumple your napkin and throw it on top of your plate so you don't continue to eat when you are no longer hungry.

2. **Smaller plates** may help you feel more satisfied by your food portions *and* limit the amount you can put on the plate.

3. **Watch portion size.** If you are *truly* hungry, you can always add more food to your plate once you've finished your initial serving. But remember to count the additional food accordingly.

4. **Always eat at your dining room or kitchen table.** You deserve better than nibbling from an open refrigerator or over the sink. Make an attractive place setting, even if you're eating alone. Feed your eyes as well as your stomach. By always eating at a table, you will become much more aware of your true food intake. For some reason, many of us conveniently "forget" the food we swallow while standing over the stove or munching in the car or on the run.

5. **Avoid doing anything else while you are eating.** If you read the paper or watch television while you eat, it's easy to consume too much food without realizing it because you are concentrating on something else besides what you're eating. Then, when you look down at your plate and see that it's empty, you wonder where all the food went and why you still feel hungry.

Day by day, as you travel the path to good health, it will become easier to make the right choices, to eat *smarter*. But don't ever fool yourself into thinking that you'll be able to put your eating habits on cruise control and forget about them. Making a commitment to eat good, healthy food and sticking to it takes some effort. But with all the good-tasting recipes in this Healthy Exchanges cookbook, just think how well you're going to eat—and enjoy it—from now on!

Healthy Lean Bon Appétit!

Index

We want to hear from you . . .

The love of JoAnna's life was creating "common folk" healthy recipes and solving everyday cooking questions in *The Healthy Exchanges Way*. Everyone who uses her recipes is considered part of the Healthy Exchanges family, so please write to Cliff and Gina if you have any questions, comments, or suggestions. We will do our best to answer. With your support, Healthy Exchanges will continue to provide recipes and cooking tips for many years to come.

Write to: Clifford Lund
c/o Healthy Exchanges, Inc.
P.O. Box 80
DeWitt, IA 52742-0080

If you prefer, you can fax us at 1-563-659-2126 or contact us via e-mail by writing to HealthyJo@aol.com. Or visit our Healthy Exchanges Internet website at www.healthyexchanges.com.

Now That You've Seen *Cooking Healthy with a Pressure Cooker,* Why Not Order *The Healthy Exchanges Food Newsletter?*

If you enjoyed the recipes in this cookbook and would like to cook up even more of my "common folk" healthy dishes, you may want to subscribe to *The Healthy Exchanges Food Newsletter.*

This monthly 12-page newsletter contains 30-plus new recipes *every month* in such columns as:

- From Our Readers
- Dinner for Two
- Meatless Main Dishes
- Rise & Shine
- Our Small World
- Plug It In
- Brown Bagging It
- Snack Attack
- Side Dishes
- Main Dishes
- Desserts

In addition to all the recipes, other regular features include:

- The Editor's Motivational Corner
- Ask Anything
- Cookbook Classics
- New Product Alert
- Exercise Advice from a Cardiac Rehab Specialist
- Nutrition Advice from a Registered Dietitian
- Positive Thought for the Month

The cost for a one-year (12-issue) subscription is $25. To order, call our toll-free number and pay with any major credit card—or send a check to the address on page iv of this book.

1-800-766-8961 for Customer Orders
1-563-659-8234 for Customer Service

Thank you for your order, and for choosing to become a part of the Healthy Exchanges family!